Praise for *The One-Hour Miracle*

"*The One-Hour Miracle* was twenty-eight years in the making—the net result of which is a deeply humane, tenderly nuanced, sensitively drawn, and brilliantly inspired work of art. This unpretentious and understated gem of a book by Hahn and Beckett offers finely honed pearls of wisdom that are at once simple but profound, humble but sophisticated, unassuming but quietly compelling, and subtle but absolutely riveting.

"Seamlessly interlacing theory and practice, the richly textured tapestry that Hahn and Beckett lovingly weave for the reader has, as its centerpiece, the 'wisdom of the body' and the body's intrinsic capacity to heal itself—healing that takes place from the inside out and from the bottom up. But the warp and woof of their broad-ranging, holistic Life Centered approach to easing suffering and transforming darkness into light also incorporates elements of choice, freedom, existentialism, accountability, possibilities, embodiment, acceptance, mindfulness, consciousness, awareness, witnessing, patterns, attunement, intuition, imagination, spirituality, vision, intention, the quantum realm, muscle testing, and energy psychology.

"Now that I have finished reading this generously accessible, refreshingly stream-lined, and beautifully crafted pièce de résistance, I realize that I will need to re-evaluate my own therapeutic approach! A dyed-in-the-wool psychoanalyst by training with decades of clinical experience under my belt, I had always been convinced that trans-formation and growth required years and years—and not just several hours. But now I find myself thinking that perhaps I have been wrong! Quite possibly by the time you yourself have finished reading this uplifting, inspiring, and hope-infused chronicling of embodied healing journeys, perhaps you, too, will find yourself believing in miracles!"

—**Martha Stark, MD,** faculty, Harvard Medical School; co-founder/co-director/faculty, Center for Psychoanalytic Studies, William James College; author of nine books, including *Relentless Hope: The Refusal to Grieve*

"With the same unflinching courage with which Freud excavated the unconscious and changed the way we understand mental phenomena, *The One-Hour Miracle* sets itself to expand the frontiers of psychology. It advocates for a paradigm shift in the field, for it invites us to think of our suffering not in terms of drives, childhood experiences, or inter-personal relations, but in a much larger metaphysical framework where the totality of Life (understood as an energetic whole) precedes dismemberment and separation. This shift of perspective opens a path to healing that defies Western rationality, for it sees the origin of trauma through a temporal lens that refuses to admit a neat distinction between our past, present, and future. Such a radical approach calls for the syncretic integration of healing techniques, from muscle testing to Enneagram to more traditional psychother-apeutic tools. More importantly, it bespeaks an attitude of mind in which narratives are not measured by their literal truth but their pragmatic efficacy. The results border on the miraculous, but the search always starts with the most immediate and profound: asking the body to share its wisdom and accepting wherever it might take us."

—**Pablo Muchnik,** associate professor of philosophy, Marlboro Institute for the Liberal Arts, Emerson College

"As yoga teachers, we often find students run into [...] asanas/poses. Typically, students breathe into them t[...]

is profoundly helpful and in alignment with a message of their book, Hahn and Beckett suggest that the limitation isn't the problem, it's the point. By bringing all our awareness to the discomfort associated with the limitation and asking it what it's come to share, worlds of healing (karma too) become possible. This perspective is a real contribution to the psycho-spiritual, mind-body aspect of yoga. We endorse this work wholeheartedly."

—**Desiree Rumbaugh** and **Andrew Rivin,** certified yoga instructors

"This book reveals the best of Buddhist psychology. It starts with explaining the key Buddhist concept of life is suffering and then describes how to become non-attached so that suffering can end. If there is one book that I can recommend that weds the spiritual and the psychological, this book truly is it."

—**Lama Surya Das,** author of the bestselling *Awakening the Buddha Within*

"It's a true joy to recommend this book to those searching for answers as to why they are suffering. These findings offer a window into healing that's possible as we reintegrate the split-off fragments of our consciousness, especially the body's storage of overwhelming, painful, energetic memories."

—**Mary T. Sise, LCSW, DCEP,** past president, Association of Comprehensive Energy Psychology, coauthor of *The Energy of Belief.*

"There is more to one's story and suffering than personal history and context. We carry all kinds of experiences, lodged in our energetic field. LCT creates a sacred container to hold and guide people as they discover and release the imprints of trauma and gather wisdom. Don't be thrown off by the title, clichéd but true. I've practiced this work for decades and can attest to its effectiveness. I am enthralled by the vivid tales that emerge from the deeper knowing of a person's body and soul. Call it imaginative, call it mystical, the outcomes can be astounding. Time after time, when a person's suffering is inexplicable or other methods fall short, the approach uncovers pathways to freedom. What a way-shower this book is, and the illustrative stories are irresistible reading! I am so excited for you to hold it in your hands."

—**Jenny Freeman MFT, REAT,** author of *Playful Approaches to Serious Problems: Narrative Therapy for Children and Their Families*

"When I first witnessed LCT, I was so impressed by the depth, elegance, and respectfulness of the method that I knew straight away I had to learn it. Now, learning has become a lot easier—the authors have set out the method with clarity and brilliance. The assumptions on which LCT is based describe a worldview that is worth the price of the book on its own. It deserves to become a classic."

—**Tony Dickinson,** former assistant secretary for health in Hong Kong government

"In healing, we deal with many layers of the body, mind, and heart. This wise book can give you the tools to integrate and flourish. Full of practical guidance and exercises culled from decades of clinical experiences, you'll find this book gives you a steady hand, inviting you to be connected internally and externally."

—**Deirdre Fay, MSW,** author of *Becoming Safely Embodied* and *Attachment-Based Yoga & Meditation for Trauma Recovery*

"I couldn't stop reading this book. Initially skeptical of some of their techniques, Hahn and Beckett fully engaged me with their integration of mindfulness and body-centered psychotherapy. Their compassion and conviction for this work is evident on every page.

Both accessible and deep, I will go back to this book again and again to better understand my own journey of suffering and healing, as well as to develop better tools to support others."

—**Judith Oleson,** director, The Tom Porter Program on Religion and
Conflict Transformation, Boston University School of Theology

"Hahn and Beckett have found a way to marry mindfulness with the intuitive wisdom of the body. They show us how to tune into bodily sensations and ask a single, seemingly simple question: 'What have you come to share?' Under the authors' sure guidance, we can use our response to unlock self-compassion, new clarity, and a process of deep healing."

—**Marian Sandmaier,** author of *Invisible Kin: The Search for
Connection Among Adult Sisters and Brothers.*

"Having practiced LCT for over fifteen years, what you are about to read is an amazing healing paradigm enfolded into an extraordinary framework for understanding Life. The authors weave complex traumas into beautiful fractal patterns in Life, demonstrating how to make meaning out of suffering; the answer is within; our body remembers everything. The writing is clear, packed with intriguing stories and boundless wisdom. The new consciousness-based healing paradigm that this book introduces is a miracle itself—definitely worth the attention of therapists from every therapeutic perspective, and for anyone who wishes to make sense of and heal their suffering."

—**Shu-Fang Wang,** writer, energy psychology lecturer/practitioner

"As described in *The One-Hour Miracle,* LCT is very thoughtful work in how it addresses consciousness, from where problems stem, and not just surface issues. When we shift to the observer instead of the victim everything can heal."

—**Kim D'Eramo, DO,** bestselling author of *The MindBody Toolkit*

"This book is written like silk; it's so smooth and moves the reader along like a good mystery novel, eagerly spurring you on. Several years ago, I personally benefited from the healing modalities detailed within it, and as so many of the case studies illustrate, the self-guided inquiry led to an emotionally healing shift. Through the skillful stepwise guidance herein, these tools are now available to a wider audience in the service of greater self-awareness and emotional well-being."

—**Peg Baim, NP**

"Joni and Andy, based on decades of work with clients, have produced a book that contributes to the cultivation of the compassionate inner observer and to enhancing our capacity for caring inquiry into our own experience, recognized across traditions as a key to reconnecting with our original wholeness, vitality, and joyful aliveness. Their emphasis on witnessing and holding suffering with safe kindness, and not pushing clients toward regression or catharsis, is aligned with current traumatology research."

—**Ingrid Hurwitz,** trauma-informed Enneagram teacher, speaker, and executive coach

"Everyone needs the light of hope for healing and transformation this book inspires."

—**Karen Wyatt, MD**, author of *7 Lessons for Living from the Dying*

"I was a mainstream MD. Then, after my son died, I discovered mediums and how they could open to unseen worlds and provide information that was undeniable but made no sense from a rational perspective. It was unclear how to bring the two worlds together until I started to witness the extraordinary healing power of LCT. I witnessed a boy with a horrendous disease gain a sense of hope, a woman with severe anxiety have it transform, and a medium with anxiety and inexplicable stomach problems have them resolve—all in one session. The information in *The One-Hour Miracle* truly can be life-changing for you and can change the whole paradigm of how to bring the seen and unseen worlds together for healing."

—**Elisa Medhus, MD,** *Channeling Erik* podcast host

"The first time I encountered LCT, I knew that it would change the way I work as a psychotherapist and hypnotherapist. Little did I know how much the work would change my life through an impromptu healing session! I read about a hundred books a year, many of them in the field of psychology. Rarely do I find one that is a page-turner; that I have a hard time putting down. Hahn and Beckett's new book is filled with interesting theory and compelling case studies that illustrate the framework that allows for deep, lasting change and healing. They give ways to heal physically, emotionally, and spiritually that you can do at home by yourself or with someone you trust guiding you. I highly recommend it, particularly if you have tried all kinds of other modalities but haven't found the results you want and deserve to have."

—**Elizabeth Bonet, PhD, LMHC,** *Hypnotize Me* podcast host

"I highly recommend this book to people who are looking for a new approach to everyday problems."

—**Sharon Saline, PsyD,** clinical psychologist, speaker, and author of *What Your ADHD Child Wishes You Knew*

"*The One-Hour Miracle* is a brilliant introduction to one of the highest-level solutions for suffering that I have ever known. Hahn and Beckett are pioneers in modern medicine, able to see that imagination is the key to a solid foundation for well-being. Working with them has led me to profound breakthroughs, so much so that I often refer LCT to my own clients. We have long needed a version of therapy that asserts that who we are is powerful enough to break through all perceived limitations. Hahn and Beckett have discovered that version and, in this book, offer it generously to the world."

—**Amisha Patel,** founder, The Tree of Life Success series

"The world of energetic healing is here, and Andy and Joni's work is at the forefront of healing trauma and, therefore, disease. I love and endorse their work."

—**Richard Flook,** author of *Why Am I Sick?*

"I've been familiar with LCT for over twenty years, and the work is truly cutting edge. It is a system that creates a two-way communication between the conscious mind and the body that allows real healing to occur in a most natural and profound way."

—**David Irvine, MD**

"I heartily applaud Hahn and Beckett for the significant healing transformations they are making in people's lives as they actively pursue their mission to help end all suffering. I highly recommend it!"

—**Irene Weinberg,** author of *They Serve Bagels in Heaven,* host of *Grief and Rebirth* podcast

THE
One-Hour
MIRACLE

A 5-Step Process to
Guide Your Self-Healing

Change the Story, Re-author Your Life

Andrew Hahn, PsyD,
and Joan Beckett, LMHC, MBA

Health Communications, Inc.
Boca Raton, Florida

www.hcibooks.com

This book is not intended as a substitute for the medical advice of physicians and mental health professionals. The reader should regularly consult a physician and mental health professional in matters relating to their health, and particularly with respect to any symptoms that may require diagnosis or medical attention.

The protocol in this book should not be used for self-help by anyone who has certain symptoms. These symptoms include delusions, hallucinations, periods of time in your life that you can't account for, and suicidal ideation. Also, if you have a diagnosis of DID or borderline personality disorder with any psychotic features, as well as if you have a severe addiction, you should *not* use this protocol for self-help. If you choose to use Life Centered Therapy, these symptoms and diagnoses require the support of a mental health professional trained in Life Centered Therapy and are beyond the scope of this book for self-help.

Library of Congress Cataloging-in-Publication Data
is available through the Library of Congress

© 2022 Andrew Hahn, PsyD, and Joan Beckett, LMHC, MBA

ISBN-13: 978-07573-2415-4 (Paperback)
ISBN-10: 07573-2415-0 (Paperback)
ISBN-13: 978-07573-2416-1 (ePub)
ISBN-10: 07573-2416-9 (ePub)

HCI, its logos, and marks are trademarks of Health Communications, Inc.

Publisher: Health Communications, Inc.
          1700 NW 2nd Avenue
          Boca Raton, FL 33432-1653

Cover design by Larissa Hise Henoch
Interior design by Larissa Hise Henoch, formatting by Lawna Patterson Oldfield

This book is dedicated to all
those who have chosen to take the journey.
Seeking a freedom-filled life can at times feel arduous.
Your willingness and tenacity to stay with
the process is inspirational.
We feel privileged and grateful for your
presence in our lives.

Contents

Foreword

The first time I saw a spontaneous remission of a serious disease, it rocked my view of modern medicine. As a physician who has seen multiple unexplained healings and witnessed remarkable before and after stories, my mission is to learn more about how to assist with these occurrences. Can we determine what dynamics are facilitating and encouraging the unexpected regression of a disease or illness? Why not use these principles with everyone? While dramatic healings may be rare, these concepts can help to lessen the suffering and the burden of disease for many.

In the book *The One-Hour Miracle,* Dr. Andrew Hahn and Joan Beckett make a huge claim. A one-hour miracle? Hahn and Beckett are delving into mechanisms that stimulate the body's innate ability to self-heal. If it feels too New Age, or too large of a claim, one only needs to look at the placebo effect. While often discounted by medicine, the placebo effect is a testament to the fact that at least 30 percent of all healing and cure comes from self-healing mechanisms involving the body and mind. Further, look at the Institute of Noetic Sciences; they have documented over 2,000 cases of unexplained remissions globally with thorough examination of the circumstances and the medical charts for each case.

The origin of illness and disease is multifactorial, and we do not fully understand it. Each traditional paradigm of medicine has different underpinnings of health and illness. Put simply, traditional Chinese medicine attributes many illnesses to the individual organs being in disharmony or out of balance. In the Hawaiian tradition, illness may be a sign that ancestors from the previous generations contributing to the soul and body of the patient are not in harmony or not "getting along" within the person. Hippocrates described illness as an imbalance of the four humors or fluids in the body. Imbalance is initiated or caused by something, and Hahn and Beckett are going after this aspect in healing. What is the incident that caused the imbalance?

The division between the mind and body was initiated by the writings of the philosopher Descartes. We have learned to use this reductionism in medicine. I am often asked, "Is this an energy illness or physical illness?" or "Should I address the dietary changes first or the trauma that led to the depression first?" Prior to our current one cause/one cure medical model, every tradition understood that the wholeness of body and mind were important for healing. Further, we all intuitively know that the mind and body work synergistically. In fact, more and more evidence for the effect the mind exerts on the body, and the body exerts on the mind, is flourishing in the medical literature, especially with regard to mental health and chronic pain. Hahn and Beckett's work involves both mind and body at the same time, the long awaited "and" instead of "or." Mind and body united and addressed in a healing modality.

What Hahn and Beckett bring to us is a healing model based on trauma as the incident that initiated the imbalance for the illness. The body can somatically carry our history and personal story the same way memories work in the mind. This includes trauma in this life as well as the trauma an individual may carry historically, genetically, (or karmically, if that fits your belief system.) On another note, belief in this model is not required for healing to occur; the technique works its magic on its own as it unites one's conscious and unconscious processes to illuminate something deeper.

As an integrative medicine physician, the way I vet new healing techniques I am exploring is the following: Is it effective? Yes, the authors bring us many stories of healing both spontaneous (one-hour miracles) as well as those that heal over time. Next, does it cause harm? This simple technique does not cause harm. We are not adding chemicals into the body or removing organs or nerves, and if too much vulnerability or fear occurs, the client can shut the process down. Next, I look to see if the modality has biologic plausibility. This technique does have biologic plausibility directly through the mind-body connection. And finally, I want to know if a healing technique can be shared and taught for others to perform. Hahn and Becket do this remarkably well. They share how to use Life Centered Therapy, their body-full hypnotic technique for innate healing, for anyone who has the desire to learn it. Anyone can learn this, so why not learn it?

I have the privilege of writing this foreword with the editor of The One-Hour Miracle, Meghan Davis-Hill. Her intimacy with the material shared by Hahn and Beckett stimulated her desire to offer her personal experience to the reader. **Editor and physician together professionally and personally experiencing this work, endorsing this work and encouraging you to read this material, to absorb it, and to embrace it.**

—**Ann Marie Chiasson, MD, MPH,** Director, Fellowship in Integrative Medicine, at the University of Arizona Andrew Weil Center forIntegrative Medicine, and author of *Energy Healing: The Essentials of Self-Care*

As an editor of this book, I had a duty to make sure that the material could be understood by the reader with no psychology background and to make sure that the instructions were clear so that any reader could utilize the tools of Life Centered Therapy at home. So, using myself as the test reader, I attempted to follow the instructions and try some of these tools out on myself.

In the beginning of the book, there's a line that Andy and Joni wrote that basically says that if you only get one thing out of this entire book, they hope that you'll get the tool to directly address the physical sensation of your emotion and ask it what it has to share. I thought about what physical feeling in my body pops up when I'm feeling stressed.

For as long as I can remember, it's been a tightness in my chest that constricts my breathing a bit. I honestly can't remember a time in my life when I didn't have that feeling at least once a day. I've always been a Type-A, driven person. I figured that stress just came along with whatever I was trying to accomplish on any given day. It was the only physical feeling I could think of when reading that passage. So, I closed my eyes, took some calming breaths, tried to really focus on that tight chest feeling, and asked out loud: "Tightness in Chest, what have you come to share with me?"

At first, nothing happened. I was just sitting there with my eyes closed, slowly breathing in and out, in and out. Impatient as any of my fellow Type-A readers out there, I asked again out loud: "Tightness in Chest, what have you come to share with me?" The response came to me in an instant this time, in an inner voice in my mind that I can only describe as soothing—like the voice of my mother who's been deceased for over ten years now. "It's okay to die alone," it said. What?! I resisted the urge to open my eyes. I mean, where the hell did *that* come from? I took a few breaths, trying to wrap my head around the message. "It's okay to die alone," the voice said again. "It's okay—you'll be okay."

My mind traveled to my four children. I had several thoughts. Is part of the reason why I feel such a strong need to be there for them in every moment, even as they transition into adulthood, because I'm afraid that they'll leave me and not come back—leaving me alone? Yep—hard yes. Is part of my drive to achieve in everything I do because I hope that my success will make people want to be around me so that I don't end up alone? Yes again. Well, damn. But what if I don't like to be alone anyway? "There's peace—you'll feel peaceful," the voice said. Suddenly, I just knew that that was true.

I opened my eyes, and a wave of peace washed through me, taking my "tightness in chest" feeling with it. It was gone—*poof.* I texted my friend, frantically explaining what had just gone down. I'm pretty sure I ended it with: "WITAF?!" That was five months ago now. I haven't felt a tightness in my chest since—a stress feeling I'd felt every day of my life for as long as I could remember. Damn, indeed.

My second revelation came when reading the chapter on the Life Centered Therapy protocol. I had to come up with something that I wanted to work on. To be very candid, I was feeling particularly awesome on that day, thinking that my life was pretty perfect—hooray for me (oh, the ego!). But then, it came into my mind that I often procrastinate working on my novels, having a tendency to do all other possible editing and ghostwriting work first. This was becoming more problematic since I had promised my agent that I would deliver my next novel by an upcoming deadline. Logically, I knew that both kinds of work were equally important. Why did I always spend way more time on the editing/ghostwriting? It was a curiosity to me. So, following the protocol, I had to discover what physical feelings I felt when I had both editing/ghostwriting work and my novel work to do. I closed my eyes, breathed in and out, and focused inward and down into my gut. In just a few seconds, I felt a pressure in my head, starting at my temples and radiating out around my head. It really hurt. *Yowza.*

I was super uncomfortable, but I wanted to see what it was all about. So, next step: "Pain in Head, what have you come to share?" I asked out loud. In my mind's eye, a scene came into view as if I was looking at a movie screen. It was my first-grade classroom with nasty old Mrs. Boatright pacing in the front of the room. I could see first-grade me, sitting at my desk clad in my favorite light-blue Smurfs overalls, my strawberry-blonde braids dangling over little shoulders. I was writing on smooth, line-ruled paper. My pencil was flying. I couldn't see what I was writing, but I could feel how I felt in that moment: excited. I was so excited about whatever I was writing. I felt joy—a bubbling-over-the-pot kind of joy. I felt pride. I felt in the zone of creativity. Then, *WHAM!* Mrs. Boatright slammed two large textbooks onto the top of my head. Pain radiated from the crown of my head to my temples, and then around my whole head. "I said it was time to get out your math book!" she hollered. I scrambled to do as she asked, frantic and doing my best not to cry. In that moment, I decided: *It's not safe to write my stories. Work has to come first.*

I opened my eyes in the present. Holy shit! I had completely forgotten that Mrs. Boatright had assaulted me. And she was still affecting me all these years later. With that realization, I made a new decision: I'm not letting that bitch have one more second of power over me. Little protector in my mind, thank you for your service, but it's safe to be creative now. It's safe to write our stories now. Once I had that thought and made that new decision, the pain vanished. I haven't struggled with making time for my novel work since.

So, what started out as an editing project for me has become a truly enlightening personal journey. And I understand that this is just the beginning. I sincerely hope that these pages lead you on a similar journey of self-discovery. There's peace and great joy in these pages just waiting for you!

—**Meghan Davis Hill,** *editor*

INTRODUCTION

L ife is filled with challenges. Sometimes, these challenges can be almost debilitating: the loss of a loved one; a serious medical diagnosis; mental health issues; a natural catastrophe resulting in a loss of material possessions or more; the loss of a job because it has become obsolete; the betrayal of a spouse or significant other; the inability to act on what you know is true for you; the pain of regret . . .

Other problems are maddening in their seeming mundaneness. Do you have to cook one more meal, take the kids to one more soccer practice, or stay late at work because the boss demands it even though you think it's a waste of time? Even if you are essentially happy with your life choices that created these scenarios and believe that your life is good, routines can wear anyone down and lead you to have a feeling that something could make a good life better.

Then, there are the loftier challenges that creep into our everyday thoughts, such as: *Is this all there is? What is this life about anyway? Why do I get up in the morning?* So many of us have spent so much emotional and intellectual energy on trying to find the best way to navigate life, both in times of challenge and in times of relative peace. Sometimes, this path feels fraught with uncertainty about how to understand the meaning of all that happens in our lives, from the most horrific to the most sublime.

The One-Hour Miracle offers a new perspective on what life is about and on our relationship to it that can give us a renewed sense of hope in the face of these challenges. It provides a way to resolve them that can lead to a reduction in suffering. It first does this through reframing our understanding of life, and then secondarily, by giving us a way to work with what we call *trauma*, a subset of challenges that is the focus of this book. We will begin with our definition of trauma, which is broader than what people typically think it is, and show you how this new perspective and its implications lead to the cessation of suffering.

What if your problems could be resolved and the suffering that goes along with them could be alleviated? What if anxiety could transform into serenity? What if aliveness could replace the deadening feeling of depression? What if chronic pain that thus far has been unresponsive to treatment might be resolved, leaving a person pain-free? What if negative relationship problems could be replaced by relationships filled with understanding, empathy, and a shared sense of engagement? What if peace of mind and a feeling of being "at home" could replace the despair of alienation?

The One-Hour Miracle presents a revolutionary healing framework called Life Centered Therapy (LCT) that is a blueprint for transforming our problems. Since 1994, we (authors Andrew Hahn, PsyD, and Joan Beckett, MBA, MA, CAGS, LMHC) and those we have trained have successfully used Life Centered Therapy to remedy the following conditions:

- **Physical:** chronic pain, asthma, allergies, Crohn's disease, fibromyalgia, chronic fatigue syndrome, idiopathic diseases (i.e., those of unknown origin), sexual dysfunction, addictions, and others

- **Emotional and mental:** depression, other mood disorders, anxiety, phobias, post-traumatic stress disorder (PTSD), obsessive-compulsive disorder (OCD), paranoia, loss and violence traumas, limiting and negative beliefs

- **Relational:** destructive patterns and reactivity when your buttons are pushed

- **Spiritual:** alienation, despair, inertia

While so much good comes from existing approaches to therapy, we offer new solutions for anyone, particularly those who have been frustrated with less-than-optimal results in the past. *The One-Hour Miracle* expands the understanding of both the causes of and the resolutions for problems, leading to extraordinary outcomes in record time through a novel way/ process of marrying mindfulness and somatic (body-centered) therapy. Sometimes, the transformation takes just one hour.

Amy, a fifty-five-year-old small business owner, had experienced bouts of anxiety for years that she attributed to her childhood. Pharmacological treatment had little to no effect. In just one session of Life Centered Therapy, she discovered an underlying fear. When she was able to sit with that newly discovered fear, the anxiety that she originally sought treatment for abated.

Bridget, a forty-five-year-old teacher, had an ongoing post-operative sensation of being choked. Her physician told her that there was nothing about the neck surgery that could account for this. After one session of Life Centered Therapy, in which she realized that her focus on the protection of her children was her problem, her symptoms resolved and never returned.

One man who suffered from multiple night terrors each night for more than seven years was able to heal his sleep disorder after neurologists and traditional therapy didn't work. An addict was able to effortlessly stop abusing substances and regain control and confidence in his life. One woman rediscovered the magic of joy in her life and was able to leave an unfulfilling job and move to a more fulfilling career path with confidence. For students and for their parents, too, an exciting result is that one student who had struggled with focus and procrastination with his schoolwork attained an ability to concentrate, organize, and perform—his GPA went from a 3.0 to a 4.0!

People have seen improvement, and in some cases, full healing of their physical ailments from such things as back pain, acid reflux, symptoms associated with allergies and asthma, high blood pressure, and even high cholesterol, in the absence of any lifestyle changes or medication. Many of those suffering with the symptoms of chronic fatigue, fibromyalgia, and autoimmune diseases have seen symptom reduction. In one case, although Life Centered Therapy did not fully cure one man's Crohn's disease, he wrote that, "It gave me a lasting sense of psychological and stress relief, which positively impacted my symptoms."

You, too, can have such results. All you have to do is follow a few simple steps that we are going to share with you in this book. And if all you did was this, we believe you may find such miracles also. Since you don't know this firsthand, we invite you to be skeptical and curious and find out for yourself. What have you got to lose except, perhaps, your suffering?

The Freedom of Knowing You'll Be Okay, No Matter What Happens

The invitation of this book is freedom, which we will talk more about later—the freedom to be able to say, "I'll be okay," no matter what happens, so that you can face any circumstance with courage and grace. This will enable you to find and maintain a sense of inner peace. Ultimately, this is what we mean when we use the term "miracle" in the title of the book. We define a miracle as any time you become freer of suffering. The dictionary defines it as a surprising or welcomed event that is inexplicable by natural or scientific laws and is therefore considered to be the work of a divine agency. While we believe in miracles as defined in the dictionary, we also know that many healings that seem miraculous are understandable when we open to the insights we share with you in this book. We believe, for example, that it is understandable how "untreatable" chronic back pain can resolve in one hour.

In many books, authors tell stories about what happened with their clients and the clinicians' understanding of sessions and cases. Very few books have clients sharing their own stories, understanding, and experiences from the inside out. In Life Centered Therapy, one of our guiding principles is that the one whose story it is *IS* the expert—not the one who knows the story secondhand from the outside in. This is why we invited the people who have experienced the work to share their stories and their understanding firsthand. Because they are the true experts of their experiences, the stories are theirs to tell. You'll see clients' firsthand experiences written in italics throughout the book.

Whatever you want to change in your life, we are here to help you do it. This book provides you with an entirely new way of looking at life and understanding your suffering, giving you inspiration and hope that you can create miracles in *your* life. For therapists, it reveals a new way of working with clients that provides seemingly miraculous results, with enough information provided so that they can start using the approach right away.

An appeal of Life Centered Therapy is that you can do this work for yourself, and you can facilitate others when they do their work.

One of the beautiful aspects of Life Centered Therapy (LCT) is that it is guided by the Self. This sense of being in charge of your own healing is empowering and liberating.
—Evan H.

In *The One-Hour Miracle*, we will guide you through a simple five-step process that will lead you on a path to healing. We will begin by giving you the worldview from which this approach is born. We will follow this with the foundational information that lets you understand why and how the approach works. After that, we will move right into you doing your own healing work. We will help you to identify the root cause of your suffering and to then find a way to resolve it, leading to a life of freedom, peace, joy, wisdom, and vitality. Let's begin!

CHAPTER 1

Evolution of Life and a Creation Myth

We long for union; the Divine longs for love.

What would happen if we could understand life in such a way that we brought meaning to everything that happens to us because we come to know in the very fabric of our being that everything that happens to us is in service of something far greater than each of us as individuals; and that this knowing, even when we are feeling pushed over the edge, can provide a road map of reason that invites us each morning to fully engage with life, no matter what form it takes for us in the moment?

The way to do this is to open to a new way of understanding life...that Life is a living, evolving being just like we are and, just like us, has an intelligence of its own. (Whenever we are talking about something as a living being and using its proper name, we will capitalize it.) Realizing and knowing this provides a way to be with life's challenges, having an open heart, an open mind, and a full engagement with whatever ails you. But there's more to it, of course.

Perhaps a way to understand our relationship with Life is to look at the relationship of cells to bodies. We have approximately 3 trillion human cells in our bodies. On the surface, you can look at every cell in the body, and you will find that no two are exactly alike, just like snow-flakes. Yet, all of who we are is contained in each differentiated cell. Dolly, the cloned sheep born in England in 1996, was a living example of this concept—she was grown from the single cell of another sheep. All the genetic information to grow another sheep was resident in one cell, proving that while cells have differentiated responsibilities, they simultaneously hold the entire blueprint of who we are. We wish to invite you to be open to what perhaps may feel like a mystical concept: each of us is a cell in the body of Life. As cells in the body of Life, while we have differentiated responsibilities, we also hold within us all the information of Life. And just like the cells in our bodies, we all look different from each other at the same time.

Life has a consciousness of its own, an awareness of itself, and an awareness of the world. To simplify, it may help to think of Life as having a mind of its own. What is the consequence of Life's awareness of itself and the world? It creates the possibility and capacity for Life to evolve. As each of us is a cell in the body of Life, we, too, are and have access to all the consciousness of Life and, therefore, we are an integral part in the evolutionary process. The question is whether we are going to be an unwitting cog or an active participant in the process. Do we also have a willingness to become truly self-aware and aware of our true relationship with Life? This is what we mean by free will—whether or not we move forward with willingness, acceptance, and perspective.

And just like it is true in our bodies, where every cell has its unique contribution to make, so, too, each of us has a unique contribution to make in this evolution. On the surface level, which is the personal level we usually identify with, we identify with our particularity as opposed to the unity that underlies the particularity. We focus on all the things that make us different from others as opposed to the things that make us the same. Our particularity or individuality is an expression of our unique gifts and challenges. Through the expression of our unique gifts, we inspire each other to further greatness, and consequently, we feed Life.

On a deeper level, which we might call the Soul level, we all have the same goal and contribution to make: accept with love and understanding all of Life by remembering who we truly are, accept that we are "Life," accept that everything that we are in relationship with is also "Life," and accept that we are in relationship with "Life" itself. What we are ultimately asked to aspire to is the full expression of our individual gifts while living through the knowing of who we *truly* are. This is the meaning of it all—the meaning of Life.

Let's look at these two levels. On the personal level, it is true that awful things can happen in people's lives. When these things happen, hopefully, we are able to bring understanding, compassion, and even empathy to the experiences. And if someone (including ourselves) is responsible for another's suffering, it is important that the perpetrator be held accountable for their actions.

However, simultaneously, on the Soul level, there is a revelation that there is a purpose and meaning to everything that happens. We are invited to understand that this is so and to open to the benefit that might ultimately come from the awful experience. In our experience, it is only when we have time to adjust and to consciously experience the personal level of suffering that we can be open to the Soul level of understanding. If we do not open to this second level, ultimately there will be no meaning in our experiences, and we will remain victims of fate. We will never appreciate that everything that happens serves our evolution and the evolution of Life itself. And we will never be free of our suffering. To be free, we have to both allow ourselves to be human and experience those emotions, and also to be open to that Soul level of wisdom that can guide us to use our experiences to move forward in our lives in a growthful way—that's how we heal.

The perspective that who we are is everything, and everything is who we truly are, has significant implications. We have within us everything that we perceive as good and evil—Jesus and Hitler, antibiotics and harmful bacteria, love and hate. Perhaps the best advice, summed up in the aphorism of Leviticus in the Torah, is to "Love your neighbor as yourself" —with the realization that you *are* your neighbor.

It follows that anything we are judgmental about is really judging ourselves. Everything we compare ourselves to is really comparing ourselves to ourselves. Everything we idealize or denigrate is simply idealizing or denigrating ourselves. We only do these things when there is something that we, in our limited perspective, cannot accept. When we learn to accept whatever *is*, we are free.

Accepting whatever is does not mean that we are to accept injustices that we see in life. The invitation is not to be judgmental, but that doesn't mean that we are not to be discerning or to take action when we see injustices occurring. Our perspective on injustice is a subjective experience that each of us needs to evaluate based on our own understanding, knowing that our evaluation may not necessarily be "right." Of course, there are situations that most everyone would agree are intolerable and must be stopped because when we have the capacity to imagine ourselves and experience ourselves in that situation, we would just say no. An example would be a hate group.

A Creation Myth

To better understand how this all came to be, it may be useful to frame Life's relationship to us, its creation, through the lens of a story. The truth is that, as in all stories, we start with a creation myth. In the beginning, there is only Life, Source, God, or whatever you wish to call it. Life is presented as infinite—all-knowing/omniscient, all-powerful/omnipotent. Yet Life *is also* limited. In its original form, there is one experience that Life cannot have—it cannot experience relationship. For in order to experience relationship, there must be two. And, if you are everything, by definition, you can't be in relationship with something else. So, while Life can know love, it must create something else to fully experience love. This is why Life, while being all-knowing and all-powerful, cannot truly be all-loving. You can be all-loving, paraphrasing Matthew in the New Testament, only when there are two or more gathered in Your Name.

Thus, Life creates matter to experience more love. The act of creation itself, then, whether Life creates or we individuals create, becomes an expression of more love. In our willingness to create and experience, to give and to receive love, we are in turn creating more Life. Life and Life's creation, us, long for each other. We become partners in the dance of love and Life. We evolve with the help of Life, and our evolution is in the service of Life itself. As we come to this knowing, we create more love, which creates more Life.

When we *know* and live this worldview, it is intrinsically comforting and inspirational. It moves us beyond egocentricity and being stuck in our parochial concerns to a view of Life as Life-centric.

If you think about it, all our evolution has been similar. For example, we once believed that the sun revolved around us, and now we know that we revolve around the sun. In a similar manner, all human development is based on the realization that the whole world does not revolve around "me." Darwinian theory reveals to us that we are not the be-all-and-end-all that has dominion over everything, but rather a simple link in an evolving chain.

We can aspire to this realization that we can move beyond egocentricity. When we are there, we can truly know what that seafarer who wrote "Amazing Grace" shared with us: "I once was lost, but now I'm found; was blind, but now I see." Ultimately, we can go from egocentricity in which we live in fear, anger, despondency, and a constant state of questioning Life and *needing* to understand, to a place of inner peace in relationship to Life. We can go from "Why has thou forsaken me?" to "Into Your hands I commit my Spirit."

This book ultimately invites you to be in a different relationship with the famous lyric written by Kris Kristofferson and sung by Janis Joplin in

"Me and Bobby McGee," which talks about how freedom and nothing left to lose are the same thing. The invitation is to aspire to a different version of freedom—the freedom to be able to say "I'll be okay" no matter what happens so that you can face any circumstance with courage and grace, enabling you to find and maintain a sense of inner peace. Freedom is the capacity to be fully engaged with Life while not being attached to it.

Ultimately, freedom is the capacity to love with all your heart and be present with all of who you are and then have a willingness to let go in a moment of that which you love when Life invites you to do so.

CHAPTER 2

Understanding Suffering and How Life Centered Therapy Helps

All of us wish to be free from suffering. What if our problems could be resolved and the suffering that accompanies them could just go away? In our experience, this is possible. We would like to share with you how you can have this experience also.

Theory: Causes of Suffering and How Healing Works

We believe that suffering arises from one source: trauma. We define trauma as the result of something that subjectively cannot be handled and integrated (taken in stride or handled with grace). This definition of trauma is not how the field of psychology typically defines it. The American Psychological Association defines trauma as an emotional response to a terrible event like an accident, rape, or natural disaster. This definition implies that the evaluation of what is terrible is external to the one who has the experience. In other words, they define trauma as something outside of us that we react to.

What we believe is that trauma is subjective and is defined by the person who is experiencing it. Anytime a person encounters something that they can't handle or take in stride, they experience a trauma, whether the source of the trauma comes from something or someone else, or from within ourselves. One way to think about this is *total load theory*. For whatever reason, an event pushes you over a tipping point. This tipping point is unique for every person. But whatever the cause, if you are unable to handle an event in stride, you experience a trauma.

For most of us, most of the time, we are dealing with common, everyday problems, even though they may not seem that way when we are going through them. Whether your problem is overwhelm because there is too much responsibility in your life and you get lost in the shuffle, because you are longing, even craving, for something that feels missing, and you are despairing about it, or aversion/anxiety because you don't feel secure enough to deal with Life's challenges and demands and can't take action, there is a way forward and through.

Let's take a simple example that we would all agree is traumatic. Suppose a man, we'll refer to him as John, comes to therapy for his uncontrollable reactions to loud sounds. When in our office, a motorcycle backfires, and John panics and cowers. Now, let's suppose that in 2005, John was a soldier in Afghanistan, and one day a bomb exploded very close to him. From that moment on, whenever John hears a loud noise, he relives and replays the earlier experience with all the fear and terror that he felt that day in 2005. This reaction demonstrates that the original experience was too bad for John to handle. No longer is it true that John had an experience; he *lives* the experience. He has lost perspective and now reacts to many loud sounds. So, all the suffering that brought him to therapy is simply an invitation to "re-member" something that he couldn't handle in the moment and thus was split off from the part of him who witnessed it, or "dis-membered." In fact, the problem he is aware of and the symptoms that arise from it are echoes of and clues to the original experience that could not be integrated (taken in stride). In order to be free of the suffering, John must re-member the trauma and take it in stride (get to a sense of peace about the experience).

It does not matter whether the experience that can't be handled is something terrible like this bomb explosion or something like a usually kind and responsive parent yelling at us or neglecting us. As soon as we encounter something we can't handle, it will continue to rear its ugly head and cause suffering until we are able to integrate it or to take it in stride.

Once there is something you can't handle, without realizing it, you unconsciously create echoes of the original situation over and over again. Why do you do this? It is Life's invitation to fully process the event so that it's no longer an impediment to you—so that you can move forward without suffering about that experience anymore. You really can leave your suffering behind and live free.

I'd suffered from a sleep disorder in which I experienced multiple night terrors every night. I was severely sleep deprived. A neurologist prescribed drugs—they didn't work. Then, the neurologist prescribed CBT—that didn't work either. I tried traditional therapy with no improvement. But then, I found Life Centered Therapy (LCT), and after three sessions, my night terrors stopped and have not returned. That's a tangible result I can't deny. Being as sleep deprived as I was, it was throwing off all my health—mental and physical. And all aspects of my health have greatly improved as a result of LCT. Basically, we got down to the root of the problem. It was something about my childhood. The revelation of it—just discovering it and bringing it to conscious present—allowed me to address it. I talked it out, and that process (the discovery and the talking through it) resolved the problem. It dissolved just like that! I couldn't deal with the problem when I was a kid, but I could process it as the older me looking back. That's what we mean

by integrating—we can handle it now, and we give ourselves the
opportunity to handle the problem now so that we can heal.

                                                              –Deklan O.

Implications: What Creates Healing
and Why Therapy Works

When we know what creates suffering, it becomes clear what can create healing. If we replay the original situation that could not be handled and master it this time by changing our relationship with it, we will no longer suffer.

Healing comes through movement from being associated with the one who is in the situation to being associated with the one re-membering a situation he or she was in. We can do this by choosing to be the one who is witnessing and currently hosting the situation, while at the same time choosing to be the one who is experiencing it. It is like a person who is an actor choosing to fully enroll themselves in a part while simultaneously knowing that they are the actor and not the character in the play, novel, or movie. In this way, we regain our perspective. Then, we can consciously choose that we will no longer be the character uncontrollably reliving the experience. We will then simply be the one who is remembering having had an experience that could not be handled at the time.

Applications: How We Can Heal
and How Therapy Works

Whenever we experience a trauma, a sensation is born and stored in our bodies. Invariably, the sensation is an uncomfortable one like pain, queasiness, aches, numbness, light-headedness, emptiness, or heaviness. In our experience, every discomfort we have is simply the story of a being who could not handle something physically, emotionally, mentally, relationally, and/or spiritually. This discomfort is a living being just like us. It was born in a moment, has a life of its own, and it is still living and available to us in the present moment. Once the discomfort has been created, it exerts something like a gravitational pull, acting like a magnet pulling similar echo-like experiences to it.

We can activate these sensations that are stored in our bodies by choosing to bring our awareness to something causing us suffering. Then, when we choose to focus all our attention on and become the discomfort, we are choosing to be associated with the one who is actively witnessing and hosting it, thereby moving from being unconsciously associated with the discomfort, to being consciously associated with the discomfort, and even more importantly, to being consciously re-associated with the witnessing host.

If what is causing you suffering is a literal pain to begin with, such as chronic back pain, then when you choose to bring all your attention to the being called "Chronic Back Pain," you will discover that something will either happen with that pain and/or other sensations will arise. Then, you continue by choosing to focus all your attention on and become all the sensations.

In that moment, when you stop unconsciously identifying with the discomfort and consciously choose to associate as a witness to it, simply ask the discomfort what it has come to communicate to you. If there is one thing we would like you to take from this book, it's this: when you have or find a discomfort, before you take a pain reliever or do whatever you can do to distract yourself and avoid it, simply bring all of your awareness to the discomfort and ask, "(Name of Sensation, such as Back Pain), what have you come to share?" This is the simplest, most powerful way we know to guide your own self-healing. When you have this answer, you'll have the information you need to begin a healing process that we'll walk you through step by step in the upcoming chapters of this book. But for now, just start to think about this first question.

Many of us have yoga practices where we are invited to observe and experience with acceptance the sensations that arise in our bodies when in different poses. We have found that in addition to being with our sensations in a nonjudgmental way, if we ask them what they have come to share, we invariably get a response that moves our practice forward in positive ways and moves us to greater self-realization.

Asking body sensations what they have come to share may be particularly useful whenever you are participating in any practice or therapies to manage or alleviate pain and where body sensations may be elicited or naturally arise in the process. Examples may include physical therapy, chiropractic, massage, Rolfing, and so forth.

Many of us have gone to such therapies and experienced temporary relief and found that it does not hold. In these cases where "relapse" is experienced, there is likely to be an energetic component, and the cause of the discomfort, even if it appears to be physical, may well be the remembering of a trauma that has not yet been resolved. By finding the trauma and resolving it, invariably the physical intervention supporting healing in the body will be far more effective. Shortly, you will read a case that clearly illustrates this point.

It's important to rule out any medical causes for any bodily sensations that we experience. Sometimes, physical discomfort is literally a physical trauma in the here and now, meaning that there is something wrong in your body that needs medical attention. Only after ruling out any physical causes for your sensations can you look at energetic causes for your symptoms. These may include anxiety (panic attack) that is arising in the here and now that may have been mistaken for a heart attack, or the reliving of a trauma in the way we described above.

It is also important to understand that not all sensation is about trauma. Sometimes we have fears that are an appropriate protective mechanism in order to keep us safe. Sometimes it is developmental. When we are feeling anxious in a new experience (like when we ride a bicycle for the first time) and have a physical sensation like a racing heart or a stomachache, this may just be a natural response to a new situation. We know it is not a trauma if we can feel the fear and make a conscious choice either to do it anyway or choose not to do it because we have a visceral sense of what is right for us. We may not be ready to navigate the new situation. If, for example, someone is pushing you to ride a bicycle before you are ready, the anxious feeling is trying to tell you that you are not ready.

The Results of Healing and the Cessation of Suffering

In our experience, when we are able to choose to remember and hold (feel a sense of peace, know that we are okay, and believe that we really can handle it) a traumatic incident, and if that incident is the only trauma associated with the suffering, one of two things happens: (1) either the problem that has caused the suffering dissolves along with the symptoms; or (2) our relationship to the problem changes to such a degree that the suffering associated with the problem goes away.

In the second case, while we may then still feel pain because of a problem, we will be able to accept and live with the pain. We can accept the situation ourselves, and the changes that Life wishes to happen when our anxiety, our judgmentalism, our compulsive need to understand, and our comparisons with others do not get in the way. As an example, if you are dying, you are able to accept the situation you are in with courage and grace. You will not be indignant at God or compare yourself with others who are healthy. You will not compulsively need to know why this is happening to you. You may still feel physical or emotional pain, but you will have a sense of acceptance. In healing work, we call this being *balanced*.

The way you will know for sure that something is balanced is that you will sense it in your body. The sensation that was associated with the blocked intention will dissipate. You are likely to also have a subjective experience of things "being in right order."

The ultimate result of being balanced may be that we can have compassion for ourselves and others and, at the same time, know that there are perspectives far greater than our personal perspective, which we may never understand. Those greater perspectives can provide meaning and some solace for any experience, situation, or context in which we find ourselves.

A Story: Waves of Pain

Before sharing this story, two caveats. First, we do not tape-record sessions, so the stories and cases in this book come from written notes and memory. Second, the stories that follow may seem miraculous. While it is not unique to have such dramatic results, it is unusual. Such results typically happen when there is only one crystallizing event leading to one or more dramatic symptoms. For example, an extreme fear of elevators and a general claustrophobia are two symptoms that a client suffered from ever since she was trapped in an elevator as a child. But sometimes, one symptom may not transform for a long time because it has so many different streams that have ultimately contributed to the river we call your symptom. We will later share a case where a woman came in because she could not have her blood drawn, and it took over a year to resolve the symptom sufficiently so she could.

The simplest way to share what we mean by "What causes suffering?" and "What creates healing?" is to share the story of an actual session that happened at a demonstration.

One of the participants apologized in advance and said that she would have to get up repeatedly because she had had a bad accident. If she sat for too long, more than a few minutes, she would feel significant pain. She was randomly chosen to be the subject for our demonstration and needed to stand through it in order to feel comfortable.

She told us that she only had one intention: "to be free of back pain." She shared her story briefly. Several years ago, at the beach, she was knocked over by a wave and got badly hurt. Doctors told her that her injury was similar to whiplash that happens in a car accident.

Even though they told her that the back pain ought to go away over time, it never lessened. She was certain that the accident caused her back pain. She sought further assistance from specialists and bodyworkers, to no avail.

We discovered, through muscle testing (described in Chapter 4), that her wave accident was not the primary cause of her back pain. The woman believed in the possibility of other lifetimes, that her back pain could be a manifestation of an energetic template from a past life. She therefore opened to her back pain being caused by more than just the accident in the wave.

Stick with us here, dear reader. You don't have to believe in past lives to benefit from Life Centered Therapy. We'll explain in a later chapter the nature of lifetimes and how Soul can come down through an energetic line, which is related to karma, or through the blood line, which is related to genealogy. But we'll also discuss how to do this work if your belief system does not include other lifetimes. You decide. This work is comparable to play therapy, which many therapists utilize with great success. As one client who resolved her suicidal thoughts and urges said, "Do I believe in past lives? Does it matter? I'm astonished to still be here!"

Continuing our work, our diagnostic system (that we share in Chapter 14) suggested that the template had crystallized in what is called a karmic past life. Put more simply, the woman experienced a trauma in a past life that was affecting her in the present. What is important in this context is not whether the past life story the woman told was literally factual or not, but whether it was useful in healing. Veracity is more of a philosophical question, not a therapeutic one.

Our diagnostic system further revealed that the woman's back pain was born of a betrayal. To put it differently, muscle testing revealed that the story included a betrayal of trust and back pain held that betrayal.

I invited her to bring all her attention to back pain and to "the betraying of trust" and then to scan her body and to tell us what she was experiencing in the body. Immediately, her back pain intensified.

I then invited her to bring all of her awareness to "back pain" and to focus all of her attention on it as though she were "back pain"; that she was someone whose name was Back Pain. She might become a person having back pain, like being a character in a play, or images might come to her, like watching a movie, or feelings and ideas might come, like being immersed in a novel. She was just to report and share as though Back Pain were telling its story.

Speaking directly to Back Pain, I asked, "Where are you beginning? What's happening? What have you come to share?"

Though she had never done anything like this before, she immediately experienced herself as wearing a Roman toga. She was a man, a general, and the leader of an army. They were in a desert.

Across from them was an opposing army. The two leaders of the armies met and decided that the two men would fight each other. The loser's army would become prisoners of the winning general's army.

The leader returned to his troops and told them of the agreement. He would fight the fight for them. He then, somewhat arrogantly, said that he was going to win.

When the two met in battle, the leader was somewhat nonchalant, inattentive, and distracted. The other leader knocked him down and, as he was trying to stand, "a wave" of windblown sand caused him to lose his balance and fall back again on his back.

As he rolled onto his stomach, preparing to stand, he realized that the other general had gotten behind him and was about to stab him in his back. His final thought was that he had betrayed his men.

I invited the woman, as the leader, to complete the death process (we will discuss this in a later chapter) and to go to the time between lives and find the souls of the men he believed he had betrayed. The leader had anticipated that the men would despise him. Instead, he found they had forgiven him. They told him that they realized he was human, and, in his humanness, he was inattentive just as they had been in not hearing the approaching army sooner. Forgiveness had come 2,000 years ago.

After feeling the forgiveness which released the unconscious guilt, the woman let out a sigh of relief and said that she thought she was done. Muscle testing affirmed this. She then said that she wanted to sit because she was tired.

She told us the story of the wave accident. She and a group of mothers were at the beach, and it was her turn to watch the children in the water. She was somewhat inattentive, distracted, and nonchalant about this, figuring that they would be okay. When she turned to look at them, it appeared that one of the children was having trouble. She raced into the water to try to help the child and was knocked over by a big wave. She hit her back on a rock and was incapacitated. All of the children got out on their own, while she had to be brought to shore.

The leader's story is an energetic template for the experience the woman had at the beach. What we mean by this is the two events are very similar—as similar as Life could make them 2,000 years apart. This goes so far as to even use the same literal word for the cause of the problem. She described what knocked her over in the desert as a wave of windblown sand, and it was a wave that knocked her over in the ocean.

The core themes are the same—ignoring role, nonchalance, and betrayal. In both cases, she was an authority, was responsible for a group of other people, and was supposed to watch out for them. The soldiers were trained in warfare, and the children were trained in swimming. She didn't let soldiers fight, but she let the kids go swimming—that was a step forward for her. But she still stumbled with her nonchalance—she failed to be responsible again. The general was knocked over by his opponent, and the mom was forced to race out in a frenzied manner because each of them wasn't paying attention. Both the general and the mother were not in right relationship with responsibility.

The mom (in her conscious mind or ego) thought it was an accident of fate. But accidents may not be accidents at all—in this case, it seems that the accident is the point. Our Soul wants to present to us an opportunity to evolve. So, we often unconsciously play out circumstances that echo events from the past in order to heal and grow.

As we introduced in Chapter 1, on a Soul-level, we might say that we unconsciously co-create these difficulties as a way to remember, heal, and grow, to master these experiences in the service of our own evolution, the evolution of those around us, and the evolution of Life itself. At the very least, we can say that the template acts like a magnet, drawing similar experiences to it. In this way, Life is like a classroom where we continue to act out and relive variations of a crystallizing moment until we have mastered it. This perhaps is a different and less typical way of understanding the law of attraction. We might say that we attract to ourselves what is needed in order to heal and grow, even if it isn't ego gratifying and doesn't seem life enhancing.

To reiterate, as this story shows, from our personal (conscious mind and ego) perspective, it just seems like we are victims of fate. So, we might say that our evolution is the movement from experiencing ourselves as victims of fate to experiencing ourselves as free and co-creators of destiny. And it is critical to clarify that terrible things that happen to a person are not the victim's fault. In the material world, the person has nothing to do with what happened. They simply have a Soul-level wound, and Life is providing an opportunity for them to heal.

It is so important to hold ourselves and others on both personal and Soul perspectives. If we were only to hold the Soul perspective, there is only one question we could ask when something bad happens: how does this event serve Life? Asking only that question without recognizing and embracing our humanity and suffering is just cruel. Asking a victim of abuse how the abuse served Life is a form of victim-blaming in the worst of all possible ways. Instead, we should strive for empathy and compassion in the wake of bad things happening to us, our family, friends; in fact, anyone.

Then, after some healing has occurred on this conscious level, we must try to take the next step to place meaning on our bad experience and ask how we can think about it in another way or use the experience differently moving forward in our lives. If I was assaulted a year ago, after some healing on the conscious level, is there a way for me to grow from that experience? Could I gain resilience, strength, or perseverance? Could I start a community watch or become a black belt in karate? Could I appreciate my inner strength—something I didn't even consciously realize I had before? The fundamental Soul-level question I'd eventually ask is: what exactly do I need to heal within myself? We are then likely to discover that the "bad" things that happened to us may also actually be opportunities to heal what we might call karma.

In another example, let's say that I am diagnosed with cancer. On a conscious level, I have to grieve—I'm only human, and this diagnosis and treatment can be crushing. Wrapping my conscious mind around this reality won't be easy. But I hope to eventually be able to get myself to a place where I can ask myself how I can think about this experience in a different way. Is it possible for me to learn something about myself or others through this experience? Is it possible for me to think about how my journey through cancer treatment could help others in some way? Posing these questions can lead me to the Soul-level learnings around this challenging experience.

If I can discover the answer and heal trauma(s), then I'll be able to handle the cancer diagnosis and treatment regimen with a sense of peace and grace. If I stay only in my conscious level of thought, then I won't be able to find any meaning in my suffering. It's the capacity to hold both perspectives at the same time (the conscious and Soul perspectives) with courage and grace that is the key to all healing. It's also one of the hardest things to do in life. But stick with us, and we'll show you the way.

Bringing our attention to these energetic templates (symptoms of the traumas we need to heal) improves our lives in the here and now. For the woman in our demonstration, her chronic back pain disappeared. As we said previously, she asked to sit down after the session was over so she could rest for a few minutes before she had to stand up again. After about an hour, she had the startling realization that she had been sitting pain-free. She would have found this unbelievable except for the fact that she had to honor her own subjective knowing.

She had the sense that she was tired of being overly responsible and fighting other people's battles for them. Simultaneously, she thought it possible that when she did choose to do something, she would truly choose it instead of acting out of subconscious guilt. A month later, she reported that she was still pain-free, and she was feeling more able to make heartfelt choices in her life. We know that this story and stories like this are real because we have experienced them ourselves and because we have seen the results with our clients.

> *In Life Centered Therapy, we're working with whatever your con-*
> *cept of a higher being is. Although I may not be 100 percent sure*
> *of what I believe, I am 100 percent sure that it works because I've*
> *seen amazing changes in my life for the first time.*
>   —Roger S.

We invite you to follow in the way of the audience in a drama, with a willing suspension of disbelief, so that you maintain both your skepticism and your curiosity as you enter into the world and the journey we call Life Centered Therapy.

CHAPTER 3

Everything You Need to Know About Why and How Life Centered Therapy Works

There are some significant ideas that are important to know and understand as we help you learn to create miracles in your life. We've touched on some of them in the introductory chapters, and for those, we feel they warrant being highlighted again. Sharing other foundational concepts will make it easier to understand the model.

Overview

Our symptoms can cause us great suffering, and, on a whole other level, they are an invitation to remembering what couldn't be taken in stride so that we can master what previously couldn't be handled. This mastering leads to healing and growth. The simplest and most powerful way to heal is through discovering body sensations associated with our suffering. When we bring all our awareness to these body sensations (mindfulness) and choose to become them from the inside out (somatics), the work becomes safer, more effective, and more efficient.

Every body sensation is a member of the community of Soul, just as we are. It is not Andy or Joni's Soul; it is that each of us is the current expression of the manifestation of a Soul. The only difference between Andy and Joni and all the sensations is that we are the ones who embody the sensations and can choose where to bring attention, because the spotlight, so to speak, is on us.

It is not the one we identify with, in our case Andy or Joni, that is the client doing the healing, although they are the ones seeking the healing. It is Discomfort itself that is the client. We talk directly to Discomforts, and we receptively listen to and share what they have come to say.

The implications of this are truly stunning for our field. First, there can be no such thing as re-traumatization because we are choosing to be the one who is traumatized, without identifying with that one as who we are. It is not us. We are just fully aligning with the witness who is holding the one who is traumatized.

Second, it follows that there is no such thing as regression. Everything is happening in the here and now, including our finding sensations that have come to share their stories. Since there is no regression, there is no need to "conventionally" resource the client by titrating the experience. All the resource that is needed is to choose to bring a witnessing function and awareness to Sensation and choose to become Sensation from the inside out. It's just an experience we're having.

It also follows that there can be no such thing as resistance or pathology. Resistance is a term used by therapists when a client is avoiding something in the therapeutic process. In Life Centered Therapy, we believe the client is just in a story where they are resisting something. And what is termed *pathology* is just more stories that need to be found and healed.

The work is very simple to describe. Just allow suffering and choose to become aware of the discomfort associated with suffering. Choose to bring all awareness to the sensation; let it share while you witness and hold the one doing the sharing. This allows it to heal and go back into its pure form.

And you will know something is different right away because the discomfort will literally go away. When that happens, either all the symptoms go away or our relationship to them changes to such a degree that we are no longer reactive. It is not a question of *if*, it is only a question of *when*. "When" may take a while, and it is guaranteed to happen.

With this as an introduction, we will now go into each of these concepts in a bit more detail.

Part I—A Theory of Life: Re-membering and the Body in the Context of Trauma and Healing

Life Centered Therapy Is a Framework That by Definition Opens to All Possibilities

We are presenting a new theory that we hope and believe can create a paradigm shift in the field of psychology and healing. The shift we are proposing is moving from a focus on any one part of Life, for example, behavior, emotion, cognition, to one where the Essential Self in the context of relationship with all Life is foundational. We might call this model beingness-based. In this model, Life itself is the expert, the person who is healing is the expert reporter on Life, and if there is a facilitator, they are expert in the framework only.

Any approach that lacks the inclusivity of all of Life by definition is limited. We are asserting that, in order to heal, we need to open to all of Life and in so doing, we open to every possibility of the cause of your problems and every way of resolving and healing them because they are all part of Life.

Our Symptoms and Suffering Are an Invitation to "Re-Member"

Our difficulties and/or symptoms and the suffering that accompanies them are an invitation to re-member, heal, and evolve. How can this be?

Our basic premise is that any event we are not able to handle creates a traumatic shock.

This shock, at least metaphorically, splits a part of us off from the rest of ourselves, or, to put it differently, it "dis-members" us so that we are not whole. So, our suffering is an invitation to "re-member" and master something we were previously unable to handle, in order that we may be able to "re-member" who we are and become whole. Then, we are no longer stuck and are able to heal and grow. Notice that re-membering here has nothing to do with time. It has to do with integrity and making whole something that had been split apart. From this point of view, re-membering, healing, wholeness, and integrity are all essentially the same.

Life Provides Many Opportunities to "Re-Member"

Life provides many opportunities to remember the situations we can't handle. Shock creates an engraving in our body. This engraving acts like a magnet, bringing similar events to the originating one, until we are finally able to "get it right" and handle the experience with courage, equanimity, and grace. For those of us who have seen the movie *Groundhog Day*, it's a wonderful example of how the protagonist keeps reliving a day and learns from his experiences, making one less mistake each run-through until he "gets it right." We can work things through like *Groundhog Day*, or we can accelerate the process by working with the symptoms that Life provides us by choosing to activate our trauma and letting it share its story, which is the topic of this entire book.

Life Is Always Sending Us Messages

In the worldview of Life Centered Therapy, there are no accidents. Rather there are synchronicities: strange coincidences between our inner world and events in our outer world that conspire to teach us lessons and invite us deeper into our healing and transformation. Often, these synchronicities may come in a traumatic situation like the mysterious connections between two "accidents."

It is also important to note that synchronicities may, at first, be completely out of our awareness. Through the development of a new lens, what may have previously seemed random may, indeed, be recognizably synchronistic.

It may benefit you to pay attention to strange coincidences in your life. They could be created by Life and your unconscious in the service of your healing and growth.

Life continually works to focus our attention. Sometimes it hits us over the head with a two-by-four, and other times it is more through a whisper of a butterfly. Examples may be when we have an odd thought and wonder where it came from, when something peculiar catches our eye, when we speak and have a "slip of the tongue," when we can't get a song out of our heads, or when we hear or see ourselves completely differently than we normally do. You will notice that we have included clients' experiences of this nature in some of the cases because it often has some relationship to what happened in their session. It's as if Life has been prepping them to do their work. If we dismiss or judge these experiences, we may lose out.

The Best Way to "Re-Member" Is Through the Body

As we have said, whenever we encounter a situation that we can't handle, the experience creates an equivalent uncomfortable body sensation(s). For example, if I were to ask you, "When you allow your depression, what do you feel in the body?" You might say, "I feel a heaviness in my chest." So, "heaviness in chest" and depression are exactly the same thing. In fact, you could say that you're not depressed at all. In the above example, the rest of your body feels fine. It is someone whose name is "Heaviness in Chest" who is depressed. You are just experiencing that person or being and making the mistake of identifying with them as opposed to knowing that they are just something/someone you are experiencing; they are not who you are. It is technically incorrect to speak with the client saying something like, "If your tears could talk, what would they be saying?" All this does is brings us into our heads. Moreover, we're asking the wrong person. It is technically *correct* to talk directly to tears or any other sensation: "Tears, what have you come to share?" It may be strange to open to the possibility that a discomfort is simply something that couldn't be handled, and every situation that can't be handled has an associated discomfort. Yet in our experience, this simple truth is extraordinarily useful.

> *The body can tell a story that the mind can't even really make sense of sometimes. The feelings that come up when you're telling that story are so potent and powerful. Somehow, becoming conscious of what you are describing and conscious of where those feelings are coming from dissipates the charge.*
>
> —Pauline L.

Every Sensation Has Consciousness and a Life of Its Own

Every time there is a situation that can't be handled, a part of us gets stuck in that moment. That stuck part with its associated discomfort has a life of its own. It was born in a moment just like we were and has its own identity, history, and future. It also has its own story to share.

In fact, we could say that we as Soul are a very large community made up of many beings including ourselves, aspects of ourselves (like roles we can play, which in many frameworks are called "parts"), or portions of ourselves (as an example, one of our organ systems). We may think we are living in the present moment because we haven't entertained this possibility—the possibility that a member of the community living through us is "dis-membered" and stuck at another place in another time.

Another way to think of the sensations is that they are a library (also called an *Akashic record*) of everything that has ever happened, is happening, and potentially may happen.

The Key Is "Re-Membering" the Root Cause

The most powerful and simplest way to heal our difficulties and symptoms is to discover the root cause—the originating event where the "engraving" crystallized. If we find and heal a later version, it is like cutting a dandelion at the stem instead of pulling it up by the roots. Cutting at the stem certainly has some immediate effect, and it may slowly inhibit the growth of the dandelion, but it will not entirely eradicate the problem. The root cause can be the source of one problem or many seemingly unrelated symptoms.

Often, people who have worked extensively in very good therapy on problems that they understandably believed originated in their current life and have not gotten all the results they hoped for, attain remarkable results quickly when they heal crystallizing traumas that originated in earlier lifetimes. In fact, often when they heal those earlier lifetime traumas, they realize that the issues they were working on in this lifetime were echoes that were the replaying of the original root cause and that nothing new crystallized in their current lifetime. In this situation, invariably, the problems in this lifetime just begin to resolve without needing to be specifically attended to.

Stories Heal; They May Not Be Real

When we are working with our difficulties, we seek to find the most elegant stories, meaning the simplest ones with the most explanatory power and greatest insight. The nature of these stories can be literal. For example, something happened to us in our childhood. Or, the stories can be imaginal (here we are referring to an *analytic psychology* term from the work of Carl Jung which refers to the "speech of the Soul"), like something that seems to happen in another lifetime where the main character is not ourselves. The stories can also be dreams where we can be any of the characters because we're the ones who must have created the characters. They can be daydreams, visions, fantasies, or personal mythology. They can be something that happened to an ancestor(s). Most of the time, it does not matter whether these stories are literally true or not. What matters is how useful they are in transformation, healing, and growth.

The times it may well be particularly important to know if a story is true is if we have been lied to and/or any time abuse is involved. For example, a woman was told that the story she told of being sexually abused in her childhood was something she made up. Then, years later when this woman was an adult, she was going through some of her mother's papers and saw that she had been evaluated for sexually transmitted diseases when she was nine years old. The woman confronted her family. In any case where a story contains an element of abuse, the person with the story must either seek the truth or truly know that it is in their best interest to let it go.

Part II: Accessing Our Deepest Knowing— The Body Holds the Key

The Body Is a Reservoir of Our Deepest Wisdom

In our experience, the deepest wisdom we can access is the wisdom of the body. We've already alluded to one type of wisdom revealed to us in the body. Whenever we feel discomfort, it is our body's way of showing us that we are dealing with something that could not be handled.

Even sensations and experiences that we are sure are only physical may, in fact, have an energetic component, meaning that it may not just be a physical problem in the here and now but a remembering of something that couldn't be handled. The same is true for sensations associated with illnesses. By checking in to see if there is an energetic component to what is going on, you can take a multipronged approach to determine what is causing your troubles. As we have stated elsewhere, it's important to seek medical attention when you are ill. Whatever its etiology, it can never hurt, and it can often help to ask sensations that are associated with an illness, "What have you come to share?"

The second kind of wisdom is that our bodies tell us what is true for us and what is not true. When something is true for us on the deepest intuitive level, we feel a sense of the rightness of it, and it is as though our bodies become stronger (which actually is the case). Conversely, when something isn't true for us, we have a sense of the wrongness of this, and our bodies become weaker.

Most of us start at the top with the head, and we believe that it knows what is true for us and can figure out what we desire. In fact, the head is clueless about these things. It is our gut which is the best place to start. If we quiet the head and bring all our attention to our gut and ask it what is true for us and then we actively and receptively listen, it will share. If we bring our attention up into the center of the chest, we can ask the heart that is aligned with Life what it truly desires and, again, if we listen to the soft voice, we can come to know. It is only then that we bring our attention to the head, which is in service to the gut and heart, and ask it to help us see the best way to realize and manifest our deepest truths and our deepest desires.

It Is Possible to Access Our Deepest Intuitive Knowing Through the Body

We can actually ask the body to be a means of communication for our deepest intuitive knowing. In order to understand how this is possible and to use it for diagnostics, we first have to understand that there are four levels of wisdom that we can theoretically access:

(1) the wisdom of the conscious mind; (2) the wisdom of the unconscious mind; (3) the Soul/Spirit level of wisdom that animates the body, and (4) infinite wisdom. We will describe all of these in detail in the next chapter.

Part III: Patterns

Patterns Are Universal Themes That Are Likely Out of Our Awareness

Sometimes, what we believe to be our problems are simply symptoms of deeper universal themes. We call these themes *patterns*. Examples of patterns are neglect, betrayal, seduction, and feeling cursed. Many seemingly unrelated difficulties are often enfolded in one pattern.

Suppose I'm very reactive when I don't get attention from someone serving me. For example, I go to the bank and complain about not getting enough attention. When I'm at the doctor, I complain that he's not listening to me or giving me enough time. I react this way everywhere I go. That's a pattern. My real problem is that pattern of neglect. There was a time when I felt that someone neglected me when it felt like my life depended on it, and it was reasonable for me to expect that that person would be there with me or for me. My mother was inattentive to me at one important time. I then became exquisitely sensitive to feeling dismissed and incapable of handling similar situations. The pattern emerged.

We differentiate patterns and trauma based on whether their origin is in life experience or in Soul experience. There are countless traumas (and numerous patterns) in life experience while there is ultimately only one trauma (and one pattern) in Soul experience. No matter where the trauma originates, it can affect us similarly.

Trauma Affects Us in Three Different Ways

When we have an experience we can't handle, we are affected in one or more of three ways: our head—beliefs; our hearts—feelings; our bellies—boundaries, which causes us to develop symptoms. These three ways are:

- *We believe things about ourselves or Life that, on a deeper level, we know are not true, and we are reactive about the belief.*

For example, I believe that I'm unworthy of love, and I feel anxious, guilty, and ashamed about the belief. At the same time, on a deeper level, I know that that's not true—I know that everyone is worthy of love.

- *We won't let ourselves feel some feeling, and we're not at choice about its expression.* There is a level of compulsion around managing a feeling. We will discuss the ways in which we handle it in Chapter 7. For example, at a cocktail party, my husband says something hurtful to me. It's not the time or the place, but I can't control my anger, and I yell at him and make a scene. I wouldn't let myself feel hurt, so I covered it over with anger, which wasn't what I was really feeling deep down inside. I used anger as a protection from feeling the pain of my hurt.

- *We have boundary problems, which simply means that we let too much in, we don't let enough in, we let too much out, or we don't let enough out.* Boundary issues can *be* about specific content, such as money, or about specific people, like a coworker. Some people have general boundary issues, too much or too little in or out, that affects every aspect of their lives.

  Let's look at our relationship with money as an example. If our boundary issue is to let too much in, then we never have enough money, always striving for more. If we don't let enough in, then we will somehow sabotage ourselves from making more money. If we let too much out, no matter how much money we take in, we may find ourselves bankrupt. If we don't let enough out, we may be very stingy and give very poor tips even if we're million-aires. What is important to notice is that all of these are boundary problems, just in different forms.

Life Experience Trauma—There Are Two Types of Problems: Trauma and Coping with Trauma

Sometimes, our problems are the remembering of what we can't integrate (handle). Other times, problems are the remembering of how we coped with what we couldn't integrate. In the second case, the way we coped may have been the best choice we could have made at the time; yet, because we forgot it was a choice, the one who made the choice to cope continues to protect and limit us whenever something arises which resonates with the original situation. For example, a child is playing exuberantly on a rainy day at home. His usually mild-mannered father yells out of nowhere at the boy, "Be quiet! You are driving me crazy." The child knows he has to stifle his enthusiasm, no matter what, or he'll get castigated. That was the best choice he could have made at the time. But thirty years later, as an adult, the man comes into therapy, saying his marriage is in trouble because his wife says he lacks enthusiasm for life.

Life Experience Trauma—There Are Two Levels of Problems: Material and Nonmaterial Realms

Traumas can occur in two realms. The first is called the material realm. These are traumas that we can experience with our five senses and are thought to be "reasonable" in rational, modern, Western society.

The second is called the nonmaterial realm. In these scenarios, while we may not experience the trauma itself through our five senses, we experience the consequences through our five senses. An example of this is a Little League baseball coach who curses the star pitcher on the opposing team at the championship game, saying the boy will not have the energy to pitch the whole game, and the boy then pitches the worst game of his life and his team loses.

Again, what is typically important is not whether the stories are literally factual or not, but whether they are useful in healing. To put it differently, if we transform a traumatic story that is causing us painful symptoms, it is not so likely that we will care whether the story is literally true or not. This is more of a philosophical question and not a therapeutic one.

Soul Trauma—The Fear of and Protection from Nonexistence

In Soul experience, there is ultimately only one trauma. We call this trauma the *existential anxiety of nonexistence*. Essentially, what this means is that if we were to ultimately become who we truly are, which is every-thing, we would cease to exist as something. Because we are everything, at some point, we realize that our essence is boundaryless, dimensionless, and infinitely expanding spaciousness. So, to become who we truly are, from the perspective of duality, means that we shall cease to exist. We cope with this existential anxiety of nonexistence by creating and identifying with a protective, compulsive, limiting identity which we call "I" through which the protective personality develops.

Part IV: Consequences for the Field of Psychology and For Healing and the Alleviation of Suffering

Since There Is No Regression, There Can Be No Re-Traumatizing

What we are about to share now may be what is most important of all because it speaks to the safety of the work. While this is relevant for everyone choosing to do the work, it is extremely relevant to therapists because it is a different way of understanding the therapeutic process. When we are doing this healing work, we choose to align with a witness and then find a body sensation that holds the traumatic story. It's like the body sensation is another living being who the witness chooses to host in the present moment. We are not regressing the client, and if you were doing the healing work yourself, you are not regressing to an earlier time. With awareness, you are inviting the traumatized one to come forth. It differs from regression, like noticing you are angry differs from being in an angry rage and trying to notice it at the same time.

Most therapies that do somatic work are regressing someone, the client, to an earlier age. Because this is the case, they believe, rightfully so, that the regressing client needs to be resourced in order to handle what may be very early trauma.

By asking you to align mindfully with the witness who is holding someone, we circumvent the need to "prepare the client" to access the story. The someone they are holding has a name, which is the name of the discomfort, until that being tells you it has a different name. This way of integrating mindfulness and body-centered therapy means that you can go into the most horrific experiences right from the very first moment of therapy without having to become resourced.

The resource is the choice to identify with a witness, and if you have any witnessing capacity whatsoever, you will be able to do this. It is, in fact, easy to do. And you don't have to titrate the experience, doing a little bit of work and then coming back out and getting resourced so you can go back in. It is like an actor who chooses to play a part. As they are acting, it may feel real, but they never forget they are acting. When the scene is over, they come back to being themselves. The implication of working this way is that there is no re-traumatization.

There Is Only Remembering Our Stories; There Is No Resistance or Pathology

There are only narratives that we have yet to understand and integrate. And there is no such thing as resistance, only remembering. Everything by definition is part of the process, and we can never step outside the frame of healing to comment on it. Everything that is being shared is the literal sharing of a story. The implication of this is there is no such thing as pathology, just stories that have yet to be revealed and healed. Pathology labels, but listening to someone's story holds them in all their humanness.

CHAPTER 4

You Can Know Your Inner Truth: Muscle Testing and Four Levels of Wisdom

Muscle testing is a way to get yes/no answers by applying pressure to a muscle. Typically, when you press the muscle and it stays strong, the answer is yes, and when it goes weak, the answer is no. We believe that muscle testing allows you to access a deeper level of wisdom within yourself—it's there; we promise! You may have already sensed this wisdom within you, or this may be a new discovery. Muscle testing in this context empowers you to determine three things: (1) what is most important to work on; (2) where the problem originates; and (3) whether you need any intervention other than just sharing your story in order to heal. Muscle testing is really simple to do, and you get better and better at it every time you do it.

Four Levels of Wisdom

If we really wish to understand why we suffer, how our Soul tries to help us heal, how we can access our deepest knowing in order to heal, and how we can open to all of Life in the service of healing and evolving, it is very important to understand the four levels of wisdom: the wisdom of the conscious mind, the wisdom of the unconscious mind, the Soul/Spirit level of wisdom that animates the body, and infinite wisdom.

The first level of wisdom, the wisdom of the *conscious* mind, is all the stuff we can figure out. If someone asks me, "What is your name?" I can easily reply, "I can figure that out; my name is Joni." This is an example of the wisdom of the conscious mind. Another example is if someone asks me, "How much is two plus two?" and I reply, "It's four."

Most of the time, we believe that this level, which we typically identify with, is running the show. We assume that the conscious mind is the one in control. But we quickly realize how limited it is when we get asked a question like: "Why are you suffering, and what should you do about it?" At this point, virtually all of us say, "If I knew the answer, I wouldn't be coming to see you as a therapist." For most of us, there are times in life when we feel like we don't know those answers—our conscious minds don't have the answers. When we feel stuck, this conscious level of wisdom doesn't have the knowledge we need to move forward.

So, we quickly discover that the wisdom of the conscious mind is very limited. For our purposes, we will give it the power of one.

We'll call the second kind of wisdom the wisdom of the *unconscious* mind. This is the kind of wisdom that reveals itself through dreams; or, when we say something that we didn't mean to say, yet somehow it seemed to have meaning. Or, when an image pops into our heads or when two things happen that seem like they ought to be a coincidence, yet we have a sense that they are more than a coincidence.

The conscious mind typically views this level as nonexistent or irrelevant, so it either disregards it or judges others who think it is significant as being weird. In our experience, this unconscious level of wisdom is deeper than conscious wisdom. We believe dreams and other occurrences on this level are like messages from our Soul, trying to reveal to us some deeper truth. For our purposes, we will give this level the power of the speed of light.

There are not a lot of good words for the third level of wisdom in rational Western culture. There are words for it in aboriginal cultures: in China where it is called *chi*; in Japan where it is called *ki*; and in India where it might be called *prana* or *shakti*. In the West, we might call it a Soul/Spirit level of wisdom, or the wisdom and energy that animates us (the body) and our deepest intuitive knowing. It's very important to understand that our life force and our deepest knowing are exactly the same thing.

This third level of wisdom reveals itself in several ways. It is the kind of knowing and seemingly supernatural engagement that happens when a mother lifts a car in order to get her child out from underneath it, or when we have a visceral knowing that something is true even though it might not make any rational sense when we consciously try to figure it out.

Everyone talks about this third level in the same way. Everyone describes it as a felt sense. They say, "I just knew" or "I could feel it in my gut" or "I could feel it in my bones or in my very being." When we speak or take an action that is true for us, our bodies literally get stronger. This is why the mother can pick up the car. (While we are sure adrenaline helps, we don't think it can account for being able to lift a three-thousand-pound car.) And when we speak or take an action that is not true for us, our bodies get weaker. (On rare occasions, this is reversed, meaning truth brings weakness.) This is the basis for muscle testing, which we will discuss in more detail in a moment. Again, as we sense that the physical and the metaphysical are parallel, we can give this third level of wisdom the power of the speed of light squared.

The fourth level of wisdom is the level of infinite wisdom and knowing. This is the level of the blueprint of Life itself, where you simultaneously have access to all the knowledge of everything that ever has happened, is happening, and potentially can happen, that ever was, is, and ever may be.

This is the level that reveals itself when we somehow know that a loved one has died, and we then discover that they did die in the very instant we knew. Or this level can reveal itself when we have a precognitive knowing and later discover that we knew what was going to happen in the future.

It's because of this fourth level of wisdom that we can get information that we believe we could not have consciously known. Remember our discussion about the relationship of cells to bodies, and in a way comparable to holograms, cells hold the entire blueprint of the body. So too, we hold and have access to the entire blueprint of Life.

Ultimately, this fourth level of wisdom is the level of knowing of enlightened beings— Buddha, Christ, and so forth. It is living the knowing that there is no such thing as birth and death. There is no such thing as nonexistence. It is the level of knowing where we know that our role is to be in the service of Life itself by receptively opening to it without trying to impose our will on it. It is the level where there is no attachment to any result.

How to Understand Muscle Testing

The use of muscle testing is like using a divining rod so we can access information that would be inaccessible to our conscious mind.

—Thomas R.

Our bodies are spiritual truth tellers. Amazingly, we can ask questions, and our bodies will typically get stronger if the answer is true and weaker if the answer is not true. (It may be the reason we are invited to sit down when someone has bad news for us that we may be hoping is not true.) Just like the mouth is a means of verbal communication when someone verbally answers a question using his or her conscious wisdom, the body is also a means of communication for the part of us that just *knows* the truth—that third level of spiritual wisdom within us. This is the foundation of muscle testing (MT). You can learn to do this for yourself to tap into your spiritual wisdom anytime you want. A client speaks to their experience of both levels of the wisdom of the body:

I'm a real believer in body-oriented approaches. It's so important to bypass the analytical, linear mind to determine what exactly it is you need to work on and what you need to fix it. Once we access that gut level of wisdom that resides in us, we can then access through sensation in the body the truth of what happened that is now revealing itself through our symptoms. Feelings are stored in our muscles and tissues. They have memory beyond our consciousness. They can take us back to experiences in our current life. If you dive in, you really open up to it, and you try to let the feelings come and images come, they can take you back to potent stories that give you those "Aha!" moments.

—Paulina L.

So, when we do muscle testing, we are asking our bodies to be a means of communication for our deepest knowing. To reiterate, it is not that our bodies are literally answering the question. By this we mean, if we were to ask you, "What is your name?" and you were to say, "My name is Sam," is your mouth answering the question? Well, not really. The mouth is a means of communication. In a similar way, we ask your body to be a means of communication for the part of us that just knows the truth.

Some people perceive themselves to be highly intuitive and not in need of muscle testing. The problem with this is that when we are traumatized, our capacity to access deeper truths is compromised because the potentially unconscious anxiety can act as static. This can prevent access to intuition.

In our experience, we can use muscle testing to ask any yes/no question, and as long as the answer is for the person's and/or Life's healing and growth, the answer will be profoundly useful. When we access the third level of wisdom, answers are available through muscle testing that the conscious mind is incapable of accessing. By accessing the fourth level of wisdom (infinite wisdom), we can muscle test a question that we don't even understand and get an answer that's very useful. For on this level, we have access to all knowing, even though we may not believe it is possible.

It's also this fourth level of wisdom that is the best explanation for how we can surrogate (stand in for) muscle test anyone, no matter where they are and simultaneously receive answers. If we practice, we can bring all our attention to anyone (just like we do with body sensations) or anything in the universe because, in the template, everything is the same Life force and everything is happening simultaneously. It is *not* that the information is traveling; it is that the information is available everywhere in the present moment. (This is not to say that it's okay to muscle test other people's business without permission. If you do this, you are bound to get the incorrect answer.)

How can we be sure we are accessing these deeper levels of truth? The best way is to keep setting the intention to be non-attached to the outcome by removing, as best we can, our conscious desire for a certain answer. Notice if, instead of staying grounded in your body, you start thinking about the desired answer. When that happens, we are much less likely to be able to stay non-attached. We want to acknowledge that non-attachment can be challenging when we have skin in the game, but keeping the need for it in our consciousness will help facilitate non-attachment. Perhaps the best attitude you can have is one of curiosity. It's kind of like reading a novel or being at a play or movie and being totally focused and truly curious about what is going to happen next. Through it all, proceed slowly and stay aware of your energy, keeping it down and in.

There are numerous different ways to muscle test. The idea in each approach is to press down on or fatigue a muscle, and if the muscle stays strong the answer is yes; if the muscle weakens, the answer is no. It can either be done with another person or alone.

The most common way we muscle test another is that we have a person hold out their arm, and we ask a yes/no question. Then, we press on their forearm as they try to resist the pressure. For most people, if their arm stays strong, the answer to the question is yes. And if their arm relaxes, the answer to the question is no. Before attempting self-muscle testing, we recommend that you get proficient with muscle testing another.

There are several common ways to do self-muscle testing. None of them is intrinsically better than the other. Experiment and find the one that seems to work best for you. The first way is most like muscle testing another person. Hold your arm out and put your other hand lightly and gently on the forearm of the outstretched arm. You can hold the outstretched arm directly forward or bend it at the elbow. You can do whichever one feels best for you. Then, say, "Give me a yes," and push down on the arm as you resist the push. The arm should resist being pushed down. Then say, "Give me a no," and push down on the arm as you resist. The arm should easily go down, as it is weaker. The next step is to ask a question and find out whether the answer is yes or no.

The second way to self-muscle test is to make rings with your thumb and any finger that feels most comfortable. Interlock the fingers of both hands so that they make a chain of two. Then say, "Give me a yes," and try to pull the chains apart. They ought to stay intertwined. Then say, "Give me a no," and try to pull the chains apart. They ought to come apart.

Another way to self-muscle test using your hands is to make an O-ring with one hand and put your thumb and pointing finger inside of the O-ring. Say, "Give me a yes," and press outward with the fingers inside the O-ring. The O-ring ought to stay locked. Then, say, "Give me a no," and press outward with the fingers inside the O-ring. The O-ring ought to break.

The last way is to set the intention of making your body a pendulum. You can do this either standing or sitting. When you say, "Give me a yes," or ask a question to which the answer is yes, the body ought to move or bend forward by itself like it's being drawn toward something. And when you say, "Give me a no," or ask a question to which the answer is no, the body ought to move or bend backwards by itself like it's being pushed away from something. It's like there's a magnet either pulling you forward if the answer resonates with it or repelling you backward if the answer does not.

As with any tool, the more that we muscle test, the more we become comfortable with using it. Intention and technique are important to successful muscle testing. Set the intention to connect with the deepest level of knowing, and that the information you receive is in the service of your/ your healing partner's highest good and Soul evolution. It is important, to reiterate, to relinquish attachment to outcome; instead, stay open and curious. Slow down and notice your energy, trying to keep it down and in.

There are also certain technical considerations to be aware of when muscle testing. Be sure to muscle test with the same firmness every time, push until you feel the muscle lock, pause after asking a question so the body has time to react, and be attentive to muscle fatigue and hydration. Finally, avoid using the word "should" as it suggests right/wrong; use "is" or "ought" instead, as neither suggests judgment.

If muscle testing is new to you, we suggest that you try it on different people and experiment with it, as the experience will vary from one person to the next. If you want to start muscle testing yourself, in order to get reassurance and confirmation of your answers, try muscle testing someone who is standing in for you (remember the fourth level of wisdom that we discussed above) and then self-test and see if you get the same answers. If there is any skepticism, keep working with it, and see for yourself what we are talking about. Trust your own experience.

Introducing
Muscle Testing to Another

How do you introduce muscle testing to someone who has never experienced it? We have found that the best introduction is a demonstration.

What follows is a script of the demonstration that we have found instructive (and fun).

1. Before doing anything else, give a brief explanation of the levels of wisdom we described above.

2. If a person has not been muscle tested before, explain the mechanics of muscle testing, and teach them how to be receptive and open to the answers.

3. After describing the process, ask the person to stand facing you with their stronger arm straight out beside them, parallel with the floor. (Note: Be sure they don't have physical problems with their shoulder before beginning.)

4. Explain that you're going to press on their forearm and find out how their body says "yes," and how their body says "no." For one answer, the muscle will remain strong and lock, and for the other, it will become weak.

5. After asking permission, place one hand on their forearm, and the other hand on their opposite shoulder for balance. Instruct them to hold their arm firmly (but not rigidly), to take deep breaths, and to just be curious, with no judgment, how their body responds. Remind them that there is no right or wrong response.

6. Ask the person's body to "Give us a yes," pause, and then apply steady pressure until you feel a lock. Try this several times. Then say, "Give us a no," and apply the *same* pressure. Typically, the arm will not lock and will continue to fall to their side. (Note: A small percentage of people are reversed so that their "no" is strong and their "yes" is weak.)

7. Tell the person that you are going to show them that muscle testing (MT) has nothing to do with how hard you press. Ask them to hold their arm as strong as possible and again say, "Give us a yes." Then press their arm down as hard as possible (grunting and groaning

as we press down helps to show how hard we are pressing). It's impossible to get the arm fully down. While the arm may begin to fatigue, they will still notice that it is locked.

8. Tell the person to hold their arm just as strong with even more willpower, but this time, you'll press with only one or two fingers. Say, "Give us a no." Their arm will relax with much less force.

9. Ask the person how they make sense of this. Discuss how answers that come through MT come from a much deeper part of them than their conscious minds. This discussion might also include looking at how our conscious mind, the "I" we believe is running our show actually has virtually no control. Remember in our earlier discussion of levels of wisdom, we assigned the first level of wisdom, the wisdom of the conscious mind, a value of one, and the third level of wisdom, our Soul level of wisdom, the value of the speed of light squared. So, when we ask the body to give us a "no," the conscious mind, which has one vote, is working hard to keep the arm up while the Soul level of wisdom, which has the speed of light squared number of votes, is trying to push the arm down. What do you think happens? In this case, the arm goes down because it is one vote up against speed of light squared votes down. The one vote of the conscious mind is very important, however, because it is ultimately the one that gets to make choices in our lives. This is what we call free will.

10. Say to the person, "I am now going to show you how this works." Ask the person to say, "My name is (real name)," and muscle test. The arm ought to stay strong. Then invite the person to say, "My name is (false name)." Their arm ought to relax.

11. Ask the person to say, "I am deceiving." The arm gets weak (no).

12. Ask the person to say, "I am not deceiving." The arm stays strong (yes).

13. Ask the person if they were consciously controlling their arm. They will usually say that they were not.

14. Explain to the person that doing muscle testing this way can get tiring. Suggest they hold their arms in front of them at a 45-degree angle and perform muscle testing by applying pressure with your hands or fingertips on their forearms.

Most people enjoy this demonstration and learn a great deal from participating in it. We recommend that you do it with people to whom you are introducing the concept.

We've found muscle testing to be a very powerful tool, and, like powerful tools, it can be used in the service of good, or it can be misused. It's important to only use muscle testing of others with their permission, and not because you are interested in information about them or believe you know what is best for them. Further, trying to seek answers to things that you want on an ego level (like winning lottery numbers) will give you answers but not the truth. Muscle testing can be quite helpful in everyday life when used for good. One client speaks to how he has used muscle testing, not only for healing, but for managing his time in the best way.

> *I had a lot of trouble procrastinating and focusing. I've done a lot of balances using muscle testing to help with that. I used to barely do homework, and now I sit down and get it done. I'm organized and efficient. In high school, my GPA was a 3.0, and now it's a 4.0 in college. I attribute that to the work we did and using muscle testing to help me determine how to prioritize my time. It's really helped me a ton.*
>
> —Enzo Goodrich

In summary, the key to successful muscle testing is to set an intention that it can work, follow the guidelines we have discussed above, and practice. Then, be kind with yourself because, as with any new experience, it gets easier and more natural the more you do it and the longer you do it.

Just remember that when you first tried to ride a bike, it was awkward, and it may have taken you quite a long time to get your bearings. At some point, it just clicks in and becomes natural. In our experience, and in the experience of our students, this is almost universally the case as you are learning how to muscle test others and yourself.

CHAPTER 5

Trauma and Protection

As we said earlier, our problems and the suffering associated with them are an invitation to remember experiences that could not be handled. To be more precise, the problems that we wish to heal are of two types: first, they can be the unconscious reliving of something that couldn't be handled and/or, second, the reliving of the way that we chose to cope with and protect ourselves from reexperiencing or having to face again something that couldn't be handled.

It's important to make this distinction because, in the first case, all we need to do is remember and be in a different relationship with the experience that could not be handled. In the second case, what we are reliving is the best choice we could have made at the time to protect ourselves from something worse. In this situation, the choice we made to deal with the challenging situation is now what we identify as the problem that limits us. We have to realize the choice, accept that it was the best choice we could have made at that time, and then stop living through that choice.

To reiterate, the only problem is that we forget we made a choice, and then the protection itself becomes a limitation, or to put it differently, its own problem. It appropriately obscured the truer self that needed to hide or be hidden behind the protector during the initial situation.

Since we never told the protector we didn't need it anymore, whenever anything that remotely looks like the original situation comes up, the protector automatically jumps into action because it believes we're still choosing to have it be there, even when it is no longer necessary. In this scenario, we have to give thanks to the protector and acknowledge that the earlier self *needed* protection. Then, we release the protector who came in a time of fear because it is no longer needed. Finally, we have to choose again to be the truer self that had been hiding/hidden since the original event.

Let's look at two different sessions that make the distinction clear. Both are about depression that was perceived to be biological. In the first case, the depression was an exact reenactment of the trauma itself. In the second, the depression was a protection that arose from having to numb feelings because they would be too overwhelming.

Depression as Reliving a Trauma

A Story: From Losing My Head to Seeing the Light

Andy was running a workshop at a large conference and asked for a volunteer to demonstrate Life Centered Therapy on them. The woman selected, whose name is Sylvia, came up and said that she wished to heal an ongoing significant depression which had been unresponsive to conventional treatment. She described her depression as feeling weighed down, helpless, hopeless, unable to move, and doubting her faith in God.

Through muscle testing and using a multidimensional diagnostic system which will be described in Chapter 14, we asked if healing this depression was, in fact, her "Highest Priority Intention" (HPI, that is, her most important goal), and we were told that it was not.

Then, as she began to shake and hyperventilate, she told us that maybe we were to heal her chronic fear of crowds, which she was beginning to feel at that moment. She said that she had this clearly irrational idea that crowds would humiliate her.

She told us that while she knew that many people had such anxiety, hers seemed way out of proportion and had also been unresponsive to treatment. Once again, we asked if this was the intention we were to work on, and once again, we were told it was not.

Stymied, she said that she did not know what to work on, and we discovered that this was true. She did not know what the underlying problem was; she only knew some surface difficulties which were symptoms of some deeper problem/story for which she did not have a name.

Using our diagnostic system, we discovered that her deepest problem in that moment was a pattern which, in Life Centered Therapy, we call a *Death Wish*. I told her I was going to invite her to say something that she might find difficult or not want to say, and I was going to invite her to say it anyway with all the conviction she could. I invited her to say, "A part of me wants to die."

When she said this, we discovered through muscle testing that it was true because her arm stayed as strong as steel when she said it. When she said as a double check, "No part of me wants to die," even though she tried to hold her arm up with all her might, and I pressed gently, her arm immediately fell to her side. I asked Sylvia, even if this made no rational sense to her, whether it resonated with her. She said it did, even though it did not make logical sense.

I invited her to notice what she was experiencing in the body as she said, "A part of me wants to die." She said that she was having a terrible pain in her neck, and she mentioned that this pain had been chronic and unresponsive to various treatments. She had not even thought to mention it because she believed our method worked with psychological issues, not physical ones.

I invited her to focus all of her attention on "neck pain." I explained that Neck Pain was holding the memory of the story of the part of her that wanted to die or wanted to complete a death process. At this point, it was time for her to release and to let go.

Talking directly to Neck Pain, I asked, "Neck Pain, where are you beginning, what's happening, and what have you come to share?"

I then said to her, "You may become the being who's having neck pain, like you're an actress playing the role of a character in a play. Images may come to you like you're watching a movie, or a knowing and feelings may arise in you like you're reading a novel."

She started wrenching her neck like she was trying to get away from something. Then, she cried out that she was looking up, and a guillotine was coming down on her head. She was trying to get away from it, but she was totally weighed down, helpless, hopeless, and unable to move. Those were the exact words she had used to describe her depression. She started screaming at God. She cried out that she was a good Christian. She asked how He could abandon her like this. She screamed that she would never believe in God again.

Then, she told us that the entire crowd was jeering at her, she felt humiliated, and she vowed never to get in this position again. She was clear that this was occurring during the French Revolution.

She was telling us this whole story in a very animated way when her voice changed, and, in an almost matter-of-fact manner, she said to us, "I must have died." It was clear that she was not sure. Why would this be so? There is a psychological defense called dissociation. One instance, when dissociation occurs, is when something is too violent for the person to handle, and they find themselves automatically witnessing the scene as though it is happening to someone else. In the colloquial, we will refer to this as "leaving the body."

I shared that this was her problem. An energetic part of her was so frightened to experience the physical, emotional, and spiritual pain of death that it chose to leave the body just before the body actually died. While that part would, on one level, know she had died, it also would never have experienced the death process itself. This is why she was not sure that she had, in fact, died and therefore "wanted to die" which, for this dissociated part, meant experiencing dying.

This energetic part of her was trying to reenact its story and complete its death process through her. It could not complete its death process this way, and she was miserable. This was a true lose/lose proposition. I invited her to help both herself and the part that wanted to die by completing its death process.

I asked her to invite all the parts that had left the body in this French Revolution story to come back into the body right at the moment before death. We discovered that she already had uncovered all the relevant final experiences, feelings, and choices that this woman from that epoch had made, so there was no unfinished business. (This is almost always the case.) Then, I invited the one in the story to let herself fully die and go out of her body through the crown of Sylvia's head.

While Sylvia told us that she had never done anything like this before, nonetheless, she found it quite easy (as does pretty much everyone who goes through the process). It was funny, however, when she asked which head I meant—the one rolling down the hill or the energetic one on the top of her body? Then, she said that she knew it was the head still on the top of her body.

Once she was out of the body in that lifetime, I invited her now to look up, and she was able to imagine Light. I invited her to go to the Light and to let it envelop and embrace her—to become the Light. With a beatific, radiant smile, she said, "I am the Light," and then she told us that she was feeling lightness that she could not remember feeling before. At this point, she was complete and gently returned to the present.

Sylvia turned her neck from side to side as people asked questions and shared their experiences. After a short period of time, she stopped and said that she was experiencing the impossible. She did not have this range of movement in her neck previously, and if she did try to move it that much, she would be in pain.

A few moments later, struck by the revelation, she said it was even more unlikely that she could be standing in front of a group of more than

100 people, laughing with them. She told us that this was the lightest she could remember being, that she wasn't feeling weighed down, helpless, or hopeless, and that, for the first time in a long time, she could feel the presence of the Divine.

If someone was coming for individual treatment, these problems—depression, fear of being in front of crowds, chronic neck pain, a crisis of faith in God—would seem to be disconnected. And each, if treatable, might take a long time.

Who would believe that all of them would be part of a deeper crystallizing narrative which could begin to explain them all? Who would believe that when we change our relationship with this deeper story, all of these can have noticeable shifts in a half hour?

I saw Sylvia at the same conference the following year. She sought me out and told me that most of the changes had held. She said that she had had an experience that filled her with a sense of hope and provided an ongoing effect. While not all Life Centered Therapy sessions are as dramatic as Sylvia's, each in its own way feels as miraculous.

Depression as a Reliving of Protection

A Story: Turned Away

Now let's look at an example in which the depression was not the problem but the "resolution" to a worse problem. A colleague referred her son, Nate, for a session before she made an appointment for a medication evaluation. The family was well-versed in multigenerational clinical depression and approached the young man's symptoms from an open, if somewhat resigned, position. What follows is a single, completed session.

Nate, a soft-spoken man of nineteen, had been experiencing a moderate depression for a couple of months during his freshman year of college. Generally optimistic, he had been feeling little sense of hope and was instead either irritable or flat. He had little appetite and wasn't eating well because if it. He woke up joyless every day and was numb inside. He said that he basically didn't care about anything.

In his senior year of high school, he'd had a slightly milder version of the symptoms that had lasted for two and a half months. He was not able to find any precipitant for either episode of depression and assumed that they were strictly biological.

Muscle testing revealed that Nate's Highest Priority Intention (HPI) was a Blocked Identity. In the Life Centered Therapy framework, Blocked Identities reveal that the thing we think is our problem is in fact a choice we made to protect ourselves. This choice, by definition, limits us but also protects us from a worse problem that feels too devastating to handle.

Thus, what Nate called his depression was in fact a choice he had made at an earlier time. This was the best choice he could have made at the time. While it was true that, at the time, it was the best choice he could have made, the one who made the choice kind of fell asleep. Now, whenever anything remotely looks like the original situation, he makes the same choice without realizing it. And that choice was limiting Nate tremendously.

Nate understood my words yet could not relate them to his own life. Muscle testing revealed that the pattern originated in this lifetime between the ages of birth and five, and that the precipitating event had something to do with his relationship with his father. Nate knew that there had been difficult times with his father when Nate was very young, but he could not consciously see the connection between his current depression and the earlier relationship.

I invited Nate to experience the depression in his body, and he immediately shared with me that when he focused on depression, he noticed a sensation that he described as "heavy, wet oatmeal."

I invited him to choose to bring all of his attention and awareness to heavy, wet oatmeal, and we asked, "Heavy Wet Oatmeal," who was also much younger Nate, to share where this was beginning, what was happening, and what it had come to share about how it protected Nate. A scene came to Nate that had been described to him previously but which he only had a vague recollection of himself. This time it came with great immediacy, many more details, and much more feeling.

Nate saw himself as a young boy in his basement with his father. It was Christmas time, and he'd made his father a special gift. He showed his father the gift and offered it to him. Nate's father was experiencing difficulties at the time and was preoccupied and self-absorbed, not in any place to be open to his son.

Nate vividly recalled his father walking out of the room. Nate chased after him. He could see with detail walking onto the gravel driveway, and his father getting into the family truck and driving off, leaving Nate standing there alone. The feeling was overpowering, and he remembers saying to himself with great conviction, outrage, and despair, yet also with a feeling of numbness inside, *I don't care!*

The numbing effect of "I don't care" is a precursor to adult depression.

I invited Nate to use his imagination to place the image of that original scene with his father across the room. It was like putting it into the past. Then, I invited him to make a different choice about his depression.

"You chose to bring it in; it was the best choice you could have made at the time. While it has served to protect you, it was a fear-based protection and has limited you quite a bit. It has generalized to similar situations. Since you never told it that you didn't need it anymore, whenever anything that looks remotely like the original situation arises, it comes back to protect you."

"What is important is that you can now make a different choice if you so desire. Since you asked 'Heavy, Wet Oatmeal' to come in, you can thank it, and then tell it that you don't need it anymore. Believe me, it will be happy to return to its pure form which is energetic and not dense. You can use your consciousness to externalize 'Heavy Wet Oatmeal.' Since you chose to bring it in, you can choose to bring it outside of yourself."

Nate could easily do this even though it seemed "weird" to him.

Then I said, "You are a pure channel of Source energy. Channel Source energy through you and into the oatmeal until it is totally infused with it, and then send back that loving protection to the much younger you. It is like sending him a gift from a much older, wiser brother. That much younger you needs protection. He only knew fear-based protection. You can choose to change that protection to one based in love."

Nate did this and reported that his younger self seemed much happier. He himself said that he felt much lighter and more spacious inside. I invited Nate to go into the spaciousness and find the truer him that had been obscured and was hidden/hiding behind what had been Heavy Wet Oatmeal.

As Nate did this, he said, "I see a beautiful young boy with golden hair dancing around, and a beautiful blue light that looks like the aurora borealis with an intense flowing white energy."

I invited him to put his hand lovingly on his body where that truer self had been hiding and let it come out and touch his hand and expand forward and back, up and down, and left and right until he *was* that energy. I told him that the truer him gets to retain its childlike wonder and grow up very quickly.

Nate said gleefully, "I feel so light." He started smiling and bubbling, and he said, "I haven't felt like smiling in weeks." He then said, "So why did I become depressed this year?"

I told him that I had no idea, and if he wanted to know, all he had to do was choose to recreate Heavy Wet Oatmeal and ask it.

"I know why I got depressed this year," Nate said a moment later. "I'm the head of an improv troupe. We had our opening, and I asked my father to come. He said, 'I'm sorry Nate, Kate and I have two toddlers now, and I have to take care of them.' And I said, 'That's okay, Dad. I get it, and I don't care.'"

"I hadn't made the association before," Nate said. "I'm realizing now that the next day was when my major depression started. Now, I'm realizing how important it was to me that he go to my opening. I made the same choice here; I deadened myself without knowing it."

While this made sense, Nate wondered about the year before. "I had asked my dad to come to my play, and he did."

I said that I didn't know why he got depressed last year, and if he wanted to know, all he had to do was recreate Heavy Wet Oatmeal again, bring all of his attention to it, become it, and ask it what happened the year before.

Nate brightened. "I know. I gave my girlfriend what I thought was a special gift, and instead of receiving it, she was so preoccupied with herself that she gave me a phony smile, complained, and walked out of the room. I can hear myself saying again that I don't care. I hadn't even realized it."

With that, Nate exclaimed, "God, I'm really hungry! I haven't felt this hungry in weeks." He met his mother in my waiting room and said that he wanted to go out for a double cheeseburger. Both left smiling and light-hearted.

I have seen Nate periodically since the session. He reports that he immediately went back to being his optimistic, happy-go-lucky self, and that he has not felt anything like depression since.

As a way of concluding, I want to reemphasize two things. First, not all major depressions are resolved in one session. It is the exception and not the rule.

Second, it is profoundly important to know which of the two scenarios it is: the reliving of a trauma itself or the best choice you could make to protect yourself from what was a bad situation. Fortunately, you will now have the tools to discover the answer to that question in one moment and begin a process of healing based on what you have learned.

CHAPTER 6

The Nature and Importance of Pattern

Patterns in our system are stories with universal themes, commonly out of our awareness, which, just like all the challenges we experience in life, create great difficulties for us on an ego level, and, on a Soul level, invite us into initiation and transformation. In this chapter, we introduce you to these underlying patterns that are thematic and mythical in nature. A classic example of this is the fictional story of Dr. Faustus, who is caught up in a kind of Seduction Pattern in which he sells his Soul to the devil in order to experience a kind of pseudo aliveness.

These stories may keep us from being able to release the blocks to our conscious intentions. If our conscious intentions are houses we want to build, these patterns are like cracks in the foundation that would undermine the whole process.

Often, when people are unsuccessful or only partially successful in alleviating their suffering, it is because the problem that they are working on is really a symptom of a deeper issue, a pattern, that is affecting the presenting problem. If they try to work directly on what they think is the problem, they are not likely to get the results they are hoping for—which is a complete resolution of their suffering. It is often because they are not working on the right problem. Patterns help us define the right problem so that you can get the results you are seeking.

Another significant benefit of working with patterns is that they often positively affect other issues that a person is dealing with. Very often, people are not aware that issues that seem different are related, and the relationship gets revealed through pattern. (Think about the example of Sylvia in Chapter 5; her neck pain, fear of crowds, and depression were all related and transformed in working with a Death Wish Pattern.)

As with any trauma, when we have resolved and are in right relationship with a pattern, our life tends to be enhanced. Let's look at the *Oedipal complex*, perhaps the most famous pattern in psychology, to explore what this means. The core theme of this pattern is: I have a forbidden desire for the opposite-sex parent, and jealousy and anger toward my same-sex parent who knows my wish and will punish me. When we have resolved and are in right relationship with it, we are more likely to find an appropriate person with whom to develop an intimate relationship and have our desires and needs met. If, however, we remain stuck in this pattern and it is unresolved, we tend to have what are typically called *neurotic* relationships. We may have troubles with intimacy, we may have troubles with authority, or we may develop what is called a *conversion reaction*, which means that our psychological conflicts play out in physical manifestations. For example, in the case of the unresolved Oedipal, a person may get sick every time they make plans to go out on a date. We may recognize the interconnectedness of the way we sabotage our lives through opening to patterns, and through identifying the theme of what we need to learn and master, this invites us into deeper Soul-level transformation.

Examples of patterns include Neglect, Betrayal, Superimposition (feeling like something bigger than you has taken you over and is running your life), a Curse, and, as we have alluded to, even Freud's Oedipal. There are twenty-seven or so core patterns that we have identified/discovered. In the next several chapters, we will share these patterns with you to help you discover what patterns may be operative in your life and causing you difficulties, allowing for the resolution of symptoms that may not have shifted using more traditional methods.

Patterns only enter the picture when they are necessary to help you heal. As we said earlier, each pattern has a core theme. If the theme of a pattern is operative in your life but out of your awareness, it is useful to focus your awareness, or in our language, induct you into the core theme of the pattern, by saying it out loud. This allows you to go more deeply into your body to find the sensation associated with your trauma. As the sensation shares, we listen for the theme of the pattern in the story.

Three Types of Patterns

There are three categories of patterns. *Single-Center Patterns* affect just one of our three centers of perception—either the head, the heart, or the belly. Trauma to the head is about reversed beliefs, trauma to the heart is about blocked access to emotions, and trauma to the belly is about boundaries. Each of these will be discussed in more detail in the next chapter.

The second category of patterns is called *Triple-Center Patterns*. These are patterns that affect all three centers, hence the name, and result in reversed beliefs, blocked access to emotions, and boundary issues. The themes of these patterns are archetypal in nature. They include themes of profound loss and violence, oppression, seduction, grudges, and blocked memories. There are two types of these patterns which we discussed earlier: those that are in the material realms and are experienced by our five senses, and those in the nonmaterial realms in which we may not experience the trauma itself through our five senses, but we experience the consequences through our five senses (remember the Little League coach cursing the opposing pitcher).

The third category of patterns we refer to as *Identity Patterns*. The universal themes in Identity Patterns revolve around a trauma that leads to a real or perceived sense of unacceptable danger, and a consequent choice to cover over or cover up who we truly are with an obscuring identity. We hid our true selves because this was the best choice we could make at the time to protect ourselves. Immediately, we forget we made a choice and live life through the limitation of the obscuring identity. These traumas occur on the material level (remember the story of Nate and his depression in Chapter 5) or on the level of Soul/Spirit. As you may recall, and as we previously discussed, there are countless traumas in life experience. In Soul experience, there is ultimately only one trauma, the existential trauma of nonexistence. We cope with this existential anxiety of nonexistence by creating and identifying with a protective, compulsive, limiting identity which we call "I." We learn ways to work with this trauma—understanding that personality, on one level, is a protection from a core fear that prevents us from accessing the freedom that allows us to live a life of true vitality.

Let's now explore the power of pattern by revisiting John, the man who had a panic attack in reaction to a motorcycle backfiring. If the backfiring re-triggers a trauma he experienced when he was a soldier in 2005 in Afghanistan where he was traumatized by bombs going off near him, then the example we described earlier in the book in which we simply worked with the loud sound (and the body sensation he experienced when he allowed himself to feel the panic of the loud sounds) is sufficient to finding and healing the original trauma. This is because the loud sound parallels the crystallizing event and creates a direct link to the root cause, which also is a loud sound.

Now, let's look at a different cause for the same problem that shows the importance of pattern. Let's suppose that John is having the same reaction to loud sounds as described above. This time, however, it is the same story on the surface but with vitally important additional information. In this version, we learn that John was not only a soldier but had responsibility for his battalion. And let's suppose that, because he was distracted and not paying enough attention, he walked his men into an ambush. And as he watched, bombs exploded, many were injured, and some died. John froze, tried to scream to his men, but nothing came out of his mouth.

In this example, the loud sounds, while associated with the bombs, are not the core issue. They are enfolded into something deeper, a betrayal of trust. When we have John say out loud, "I betrayed a trust," he is likely to find different sensations than if he were just the soldier hearing the bombs. Instead of having just a tight chest, he may feel a constriction in his throat and pain in his foot. Dropping into all these sensations, John is likely to open to a broader story than just the bombs going off.

If we have John bring all of his attention to and become "Throat Closing Up" and "Pain in Foot," he might share that he was leading his men and got distracted. As he walked them into an ambush and as bombs and grenades were going off, he watched as many of them died. He was feeling tremendous guilt about how he had not paid enough attention to all of the little details that might have given him a clue to the ambush. He was hit by shrapnel in the foot and felt a sense of relief. He felt he ought to be punished, and he felt that this would get him out of the war and any possibility of having to continue to lead. Finding all of this additional information, John is more likely to get a better result regarding his panic attacks. He may also get a result that has an impact on many other seemingly unrelated symptoms.

These seemingly unrelated symptoms could include attention deficit disorder (ADD) with extreme guilt associated with it, obsessive compulsive disorder (OCD) with a sense that mistakes always result in catastrophe, chronic pain in his foot that has no apparent physiological cause, a sense of shooting himself in the foot whenever any opportunities for leadership arise, and many more symptoms and limiting beliefs. John might also face an inability to feel/express emotions and all kinds of problems around boundaries and responsibility. By helping John resolve his extreme guilt around the betrayal of trust while still taking responsibility for what happened, it's possible that all of these symptoms may resolve. Remorse may replace regret, and he may find a way to heal and grow. And backfiring motorcycles won't cause him to panic anymore.

In our graduate training, if someone had come in with all these seemingly unrelated symptoms and had done a lot of work on all of them in a variety of different ways with no improvement, we certainly would have felt that our hands were full. But we feel very differently today. We know from personal experience that healing multiple, seemingly unrelated problems is possible when we open to the possibility that they are enfolded into one narrative.

Many other systems and frameworks also discuss patterns. The most well-known of these are Jungian character archetypes and systems that focus on traumas around roles. For example, we can be traumatized around the role of a Ruler, a Caregiver, a Lover, a Jester, a Healer, a Protector —the list of such roles is endless. We don't spell out all the possible roles in this book. This is because, often, what we find is that relational patterns can be more dynamic and specific than patterns based in role. For example, it is much more powerful to know that a Ruler betrayed his trust with his people and focus on the betrayal element than on the Ruler element. Nonetheless, sometimes the trauma around role is paramount, and we can ask if we are to work specifically there.

Finally, just remember that the whole point of patterns is to give you every opportunity to heal. Opening to patterns by opening to all possibilities of what may be causing your suffering can provide you with valuable insight that could help you on your healing journey.

Identifying patterns that are operative in your life can deepen your understanding of what motivates you and others. In the upcoming chapters, we will describe the categories of patterns, the typical ways they may show up in your life, and the core experience of each pattern. You can use this information to lead you to your own story—and perhaps to healing.

CHAPTER 7

Single-Center Patterns: Healing Our Minds, Hearts, and Bodies

We all have three main centers of perception: the head, the heart, and the belly. The reason we use centers as an organizing principle in Life Centered Therapy is that everybody understands what they mean: the head is about beliefs, the heart is about emotions, and the belly is about boundaries and the capacity to act.

Head Center—Reversed Beliefs

The head center concerns beliefs. When our head center is balanced, what we believe to be true and what we know on a deeper level to be the truth are totally aligned, and we have no anxiety about the truth. When we have had a shock to the head center, our beliefs limit us, and we call them *reversed* or conflicted. A reversed belief occurs when you believe something, which on a deeper level you know is not true, and you have anxiety and self-judgment in the face of the belief. Reiterating the example we gave in Chapter 3, suppose you believed that you were unworthy of love. Then you realized, on a deeper level, that everyone is worthy of love. Yet you still didn't believe that *you* were worthy of love, and you felt anxiety, guilt, and/or shame because of your belief.

There are a limitless number of possible reversed beliefs. We know, however, that by definition, the problem is not the belief itself. It is the anxiety and self-judgment we experience *about* the belief. When we are balanced about our beliefs, it's not the belief itself that changes; it's our self-judgment. And with the letting go of self-judgment, an amazing thing happens to the belief. It changes into a higher, and, therefore, different nature, in much the same way that the alchemists taught that lead can turn into gold.

What do we mean by this? Our belief that we are unworthy of love may transform into a profound sense of humility. This humility might be the exact antidote we need for our arrogance and/or open us to a deeper sense of gratitude about the unconditional love we receive from Source despite our own sense of unworthiness. When we can grieve our sense of limitation and then let it go, we discover the deeper truth. Understanding limiting beliefs ought to help you when you are doing your own healing work later in the book.

For now, just keep in mind that when dealing with a limiting belief, we do not deny the belief. We accept the belief as our truth and, by being in a different relationship with it, we also accept ourselves. Let's explore what happens if we don't do this and instead try to use an affirmation to deny the belief. For example, in this case, let's suppose we keep affirming over and over again, "I am worthy of love." Typically, two things result from this. When we try to convince ourselves that that we are worthy of love, the belief about unworthiness often takes a stronger foothold. Second, we will be lying to ourselves and not accepting the part of us who truly believes that we're unworthy of love. The result of all of this is that it just makes our suffering worse. This is because we are not honoring the experience of the part of ourselves that truly believes we are unworthy.

Now let's suppose that we accept the part of ourselves who believes that it is unworthy of love. Immediately, it starts to settle down. It feels held and accepted. And with this acceptance, it immediately begins to transform. This is why there is an affirmation for this part of ourselves. The affirming practice includes the following "new" belief: "Even though I believe I am unworthy of love, I deeply and profoundly love, accept, and respect myself." We honor the belief, and we do this with self-acceptance. Later, we will discuss circumstances in which it is important to let go of beliefs (think of Nate in Chapter 5).

Heart Center— Fear of Experiencing Feelings

The heart center concerns feelings. When the heart center is balanced, we allow ourselves to experience whatever feelings we are having to their appropriate degree, in their appropriate context, and we are at choice about expressing those feelings. Let's suppose that I'm your teacher, and I do something that makes you angry. If your heart center is balanced, you will be aware that you are angry at me, but you will not be projecting some earlier situation onto me and you will be able to decide in what context it would be best to share that anger, if at all.

When we have a shock to the heart center, we are unable to experience our feelings to the appropriate degree in the appropriate context, and we are not at choice about how we express our emotions. As a result, we do one or more of three things: (1) we deny our feeling altogether; (2) we displace our feeling; and/or (3) we transform our feeling into a different feeling state.

Let's go back to our example about anger. If you are shocked regarding this feeling, you could respond in the following ways: (1) you might not even consciously know that you are feeling angry (at which point you are likely to turn it into some other symptom(s); (2) you might take your anger out on somebody or something else, or, you might have an overly strong reaction to me because of something else that had made you angry before; and/or (3) you could transform your anger into a different feeling state. For example, you might start crying and say you are hurt, you might start inappropriately smiling in order to avoid feeling angry, or you might withdraw.

It's not only negative feelings that we can feel scared about. For some of us, some of the time, we can be afraid of experiencing positive feelings as well. Some of us can be afraid to experience joy or pleasure because they have been associated with shock or judgment in our past. We offer, for your consideration, a list of nine basic feelings that people often fear experiencing: anger, sadness, fear, peace, joy, empowerment, frustration, shame, or guilt.

Understanding blocked access to emotions ought to help you when you are doing your own healing work later in the book. That's so that you can allow yourself to experience whatever feelings you are having to their appropriate degree, in their appropriate context, and then have the choice to express or not to express those feelings later.

For now, just keep in mind that when dealing with a Single-Center Pattern of the heart, you will begin with: "I am afraid to experience/express (feeling) because . . ."

Belly Center—
Boundary Problems

The belly center concerns boundaries. When the belly center is balanced, we are "the captain of our own ship." We get to choose what and how much to let in, and what and how much to let out. We can take right actions, considering both our own needs and the needs of others. When our boundaries are balanced, we call them *permeable*. When they are out of balance, we can say that they are either too *porous* (we're letting too much in or out) and/or too *rigid* (we aren't letting enough in or out).

We can assess our boundaries in many areas. In the broadest area, we can discover the degree of permeability of what we call our general boundaries. If there's a big shock, our boundaries tend to be unbalanced with everything.

We can also assess the degree of our boundaries to particular individuals and/or groups and with many content areas, which include and are not limited to: social, sexual, self-preservation, intimacy, family, mental, emotional, physical, spiritual, auditory, kinesthetic, visual, extra-sensory perception, financial (money), work, therapeutic, and authority.

An example of our boundaries being out of balance with a particular person might look like the following. Let's suppose you're at a party, and someone who you never met before walks into the room. You have a different response to this person than everyone else, either feeling that you have to cling to this person or, conversely, to get as far away from this person as possible.

Boundary issues can also arise in particular content areas like money, as we described in Chapter 3. If we compulsively let in too much, we may have to continue to make money at the expense of everything else. If we compulsively don't let in enough, we may never have the resources we need. If we compulsively don't let out enough, we might be very rich and very miserly when it comes to sharing. If we compulsively let out too much, we may give away everything, even when we have responsibilities.

Let's take another example from psychology. A shock around a therapist's therapeutic boundaries could manifest in one or more of four ways: (1) we might take on our clients' problems and eventually burn out because we let too much in; (2) we might not let our clients affect us enough and lack true empathy because we don't let enough in; (3) we might overshare with our clients about our own lives because we like to talk about ourselves for our own ego gratification, and in that case, we let out too much; or (4) in those circumstances in which our clients truly need human contact, and we don't provide it because we are hiding behind a persona (mask) of professionalism, we don't let enough out.

Whenever we want anything for or from our clients other than the relieving of suffering, we have a boundary problem. It is not our place to try to take away a client's pain or tell them how to run their lives. If we have a compulsion to do these, it is an indication that we are too uncomfortable with feeling powerless, or with needing their approval, or with our own insecurity.

Understanding boundary issues ought to help you when you are doing your own healing work later in the book. For now, just keep in mind that the inducting statement for the Single-Center Pattern of the Belly is: "I am afraid to be at choice about (boundary) because..."

CHAPTER 8

Triple-Center Patterns in the Material Realms: Healing Mythic Stories

Now we are going to bring our attention to certain themes that come up repeatedly, both in myth and in everyday life. What we have learned is that often, when people have come in with difficulties, the difficulties they want to work on may not be the real issue that needs their attention. They may be symptoms of some deeper theme that may be out of their awareness and is likely to be one of the patterns that we are about to share.

Triple-Center Patterns (TCP) are traumatic stories that affect all three centers and therefore can create reversed beliefs (remember, this is when you believe something even though on a deeper level you know this is not true, and you have anxiety and self judgment in the face of the belief), fear of experiencing feelings, and boundary problems. The key to the TCPs is that there is typically one core-limiting experience, which is the doorway into the whole pattern. Some of these core-limiting experiences include, for example, "A part of me wants to die," (Death Wish Pattern); or "I have betrayed," (Wounded Pattern). These patterns significantly impact our lives physically, emotionally, mentally, relationally, and spiritually.

These stories come in two realms: material and nonmaterial. In the material realm, which makes up the world of our daily lives in the present, we can experience a trauma through our five senses. These trauma stories fit into what is generally perceived to be Western reality, even if the stories take place in the imaginal/other lifetimes.

There are several ways to work with patterns for your own healing. The first is to use them as we do with our clients, which is to incorporate them into the protocol that we share in Chapter 14, using muscle testing to determine which of the patterns, if any, are operative in your life and could use your attention. Another very useful way to work with patterns is to bring your attention to these patterns in a free-flowing way and just see where your attention goes. You may find that you have a sense about what you may need to work with.

Finally, it can be useful to see what patterns you are particularly reactive to. When you are reading about them, sensations may arise. These may be specific sensations like pain, queasiness or tightness, or a general sense of agitation and discomfort, or it may even be that you get sleepy and find it hard to focus. If you do get sleepy, sleepiness is a sensation that is associated with the trauma itself. And you have to bring your attention to sleepiness as a sensation just as you would with other sensations. In fact, if you are reactive enough, you may not want to read about the pattern at all. In this case, focus on your desire to avoid the pattern and the core theme of the pattern and notice any sensations that arise. Any of these can help you discover what is most calling for your attention in your healing, leading you to acknowledge exactly what is going on.

With this as an introduction, let's explore patterns in more depth. Many of them are already in the book in the form of cases, so you've already been introduced to them. In our experience, certain patterns arise more than others. In this chapter, we are sharing the eight most commonly seen patterns in people's healing journeys. The other eight less commonly seen patterns which, if operative in your life, are still very significant and are shared in the Appendix.

For each of the patterns, we have included in italics the *inducting* statement of the pattern. By this, we mean the statement you are invited to say out loud to activate the trauma in your body associated with the core experience of the pattern. The activation of the trauma in your body allows the sensation that holds the story to surface.

Split/Multiple Pattern

We start our journey into patterns with Splits. Splits are perhaps the most fundamental of all patterns because no matter what trauma happens to us, the traumatized part essentially splits off from the rest of us. In the case of a Split, the lingering symptom is this sense of being split, while with other patterns, the primary symptoms are different. The theme of the pattern gives a hint about the symptom one is likely to be dealing with. So, if your primary issue is feeling like, "I can't think," or "I just don't feel like I'm all here," working with a Split Pattern may just be what you need.

INDUCTING STATEMENT • *A part of me is missing. / I am not all here. / I don't have all of my energy. / Part of me feels disconnected from another part of me. / I feel fragmented.*

Splits or multiples result from a trauma that leads to a sense of internal fragmentation—we can feel broken up. We call it a Split when the fragmentation results in two parts and a Multiple when there are more than two parts. In a trauma that results in a Split, some aspect of us experiences the pain of a situation as too much to bear, and this part of us splits off or *dissociates*, and we are no longer able to access that part of ourselves. Or, a Split can manifest as different aspects of ourselves being isolated from one another. For example, if our head splits off from our body, we may take action in the world without thinking first; conversely, we might do a great deal of thinking and never take action. In the case of a left side–right side of the body Split, we may not be able to focus on details in the context of a larger picture, or conversely only be able to focus on the big picture without consideration for the details. Splits can also manifest as splits between different aspects of ourselves. Two good examples are that our sexuality can be split off from our heart, and our capacity for willing action can be split off from our vision, both of which can create challenges in our lives. When our sexuality splits off from our heart, we will not be able to have sex as an expression of love, or the reverse; when we love someone, we won't want to express it sexually. This can explain why some people seem to only have great sex when they have a one-night stand.

A Case: Sharing Yourself

Robert, a forty-five-year-old teacher, was married with children and felt that his life was overwhelming. He had many intentions for our therapeutic work. Mostly, he wished to clear his writer's block in the publish-or-perish world of academia. On a more personal level, he wished to improve his relationship with his wife. He felt passively reactive to her and withheld information from her believing she would attack him, and he would be unable to protect himself. He wondered if his difficulties with premature ejaculation, which he wished to transform, were related to his fear of asserting himself. In this session, we discovered the premature ejaculation, passivity, and writer's block all had the structure of a Split.

As soon as we uncovered the pattern, Robert said he could feel a jagged left/right Split in his body. He said, "They almost feel like they are different fields of energy; it's just to the right of my center. I have to choose to put my consciousness in one or the other. I feel like I'm being pulled apart, and the parts feel very different from each other. I am being pulled to be one or the other, and I can't do anything. . .This feels visceral, and I'm feeling a pain in my genitals. I'm feeling impotent. . .Oh my God; I've been cut! I've been castrated, and I'm being drawn and quartered." He started to weep. Then he said, "I know why this happened. As a teacher, I was sharing my writings with students about forbidden sexual practices. I told them to keep this a secret yet one of them told their parents. The parents reported me to the authorities which led to my death." After a moment, he stopped and said, "I think we are done."

Our muscle testing confirmed that our work was, in fact, completed, and Robert said he did feel different in his body. In this case, finding the story was all the intervention Robert needed to balance the traumatic block. Robert said that it made sense of why he had trouble publishing and why he had sexual issues as well as difficulty being assertive with his wife. Robert expressed skepticism about whether this healing session would make any difference in his life. But he reported several weeks later that he was finding it easier to contain his sexual energy, that he did notice a change in his "lack of staying power, lack of control, and lack of choice." He also noticed that he was taking more initiative in disciplining himself around writing. He attributed these changes to his prior session.

Power Pattern

Have you ever had a fear of speaking up to those who you perceive have authority, even if you feel your rights have been violated? Sometimes we just need to choose to find our voice, while at other times, we may be blocked from finding our voice because of a trauma; this is called a Power Pattern.

INDUCTING STATEMENT • *I spoke/acted on my truth, and I was oppressed/ostracized/silenced because of it.*

Power Patterns result from a trauma when you spoke or acted on your truth, and you were oppressed/ostracized/silenced/killed for this action by someone who had power over you. Often those who carry this pattern were and/or are part of a marginalized group based on gender, class, religion, sexuality, race. Or it may be seen in those who are at the center of these groups who stand up for those in the periphery—and pay the consequences. The effect of the trauma is that it destroys your ability to access your own power and have agency in the world.

When we are in right relationship with power, we know hierarchically who has the power and how it can shift and can act accordingly. We can own our power, understand the consequences of our actions, and make the best choices given our understanding. Some true-life examples:

- A male teacher salaciously told his seventeen-year-old female student that he liked watching her walk. She immediately knew in that moment that the power differential had changed, and that if she spoke up, he would get into a lot of trouble. Knowing this, she was able to tell him to "F... off." He never bothered her again.

- A young professional in her early twenties was assigned a position of responsibility in a manufacturing facility where no women had worked before. When she walked into her new boss's office, he had pictures of nudes on his walls. She told him she wanted him to take them down because it undermined her respect in the workplace. He said to her, "You going to make me?" in a threatening manner. Once again, recognizing the shifting power, she was able to say to him, "You have a choice: you can take them down yourself, or we can go to HR." Suffice it to say, he took them down and even gained a grudging respect for her.

I'm an openly gay man. Growing up in the time period that I did, there were many misconceptions about homosexuals. I was gay-bashed many times and bullied many times. I grew up in the Catholic Church and was told by authority figures that homosexuals burn in hell. I was also raped. Through LCT, I discovered that I had internalized the homophobia and ended up feeling "less than." It's not something that traditional therapy had ever addressed with me. Now, I'm moving from being unapologetically open to being proud by combatting that internalized homophobia that has kept me stuck in my life.

—Alex T.

When this theme is operative in your life, it can generate a lot of difficulties, which all spring from a core of either having a fear of speaking or acting on your truth and/or compulsively doing so without any appreciation or concern for the consequences. As an example, it can explain why on one level seemingly powerful, financially secure women are sometimes unable to speak up to men who request sexual favors. Conversely, an example may be a woman who has a very dear and long-lasting friendship with a man at work, who one day tells her a joke that insults her sensibilities. Instead of speaking to him about it, she reports him to HR and asks that he be fired.

When there is a Power Pattern, typically the first stage is disassociation with consequent denial, craving, terror, or impotent rage. The first step toward healing is owning of anger and any other feelings that are directed at the perpetrator. Next, there is a recognition of the feelings the client has toward themselves, particularly anger for letting it happen. Working through all of these leads to freedom and reintegration of power.

A Case: Seeing a Way Forward

Marybeth came to therapy because she was having a hard time talking to her husband about premonitions she was having. When she seemed agitated to him and he asked her what was going on, she found herself lying to him. This was very upsetting to her because they both so valued transparency in their relationship. Dropping into the sensation associated with this, she found a karmic story where she had been denounced for being a witch and was killed for being threatening to those in power. Realizing that premonitions were witch-like, she felt like she understood why she needed to "protect" herself from her husband. It was an irrational outgrowth of the story she had found. Her fear that he would feel threatened and abandon her if she shared these "forbidden" ideas with him dissolved in that moment.

Death Wish Pattern

Do you have inexplicable constant fatigue? Or, a sense that "I just want to get out of here"? Or, a passing sense that seems to come from out of nowhere that you wish you were dead? You may be suffering from a pattern we call a Death Wish, where a *part* of you experiences, *I want to die*. On hearing this, it may absolutely resonate, although you are not sure why, or it may not resonate at all. If it doesn't resonate at all, have you gotten into many accidents? Do you catch every illness that goes around? These may be the ways it shows up in your life. In our experience, virtually everybody we see early on runs into a Death Wish because all of us have had experiences that, even if it is just for a moment, make us want to die, or, just as likely, traumatic deaths from another lifetime that we couldn't handle. In either of these moments, a Death Wish forms. And of course, the part of you that wants to die sabotages the parts that want you to get better. The part of you that wants to die is just trying to heal in the only way it knows how. When we help that part heal, miracles can occur.

INDUCTING STATEMENT • *A part of me wants to die. /A part of me wishes I was dead. /Someone who is supposed to love me wants me dead, and in order to receive their love, a part of me has to die.*

A Death Wish pattern is present when some part of a person wants to die. If the root cause is in this lifetime, it typically results from one of two situations: (1) something so terrible happened that a part of the person wishes to be dead; or (2) a parent who cannot own something about themselves, projects this trait or behavior onto the child, and then judges the child. The child, experiencing the judgment, feels unable to hold it and feels that they have to destroy that aspect of themselves that they have unknowingly taken on, in order to be in their parent's good graces. In the field of psychology, we call this *projective identification.*

If the Death Wish Pattern results from a past-life/imagined experience, it typically results from one of two situations: (1) something so terrible happened that a part of the person wishes to be dead; or (2) the person experienced a death so traumatic that part of the person dissociated at the time of death and does not know that s/he/they has died. This part is still trying to complete the death process in this lifetime. The way to heal the part that wants to die is to facilitate its going through its own death process.

A Death Wish Pattern can manifest as mental hopelessness, suicidal intentions, emotional despair, depression, and/or physical illness. It can also play out in several other ways, such as a tendency to destroy relationships, a tendency to have frequent accidents, and a feeling of disconnection from Source.

If present and causing symptoms, a Death Wish Pattern is almost always the most important thing to work on. It often appears in the first session with a new client who has this pattern. If a significant part of the client wants to die, that part will sabotage balancing other patterns. Sometimes, however, a Death Wish may be deeply layered in the client's psyche, and other patterns may need to be balanced first.

There are three core beliefs that may be active in a person with a Death Wish: (1) a part of me wants to die; (2) a part of me wishes I was dead; and (3) someone who is supposed to love me wants me dead; to receive their love, a part of me has to die.

A Part of Me Wants to Die

This is always true in a Death Wish Pattern and clearly confirms that this pattern is actively sabotaging the person's intention to heal. There may be no felt sense of wanting to die until the person's attention is brought to this experience. Often, when asked if they have a Death Wish, they do feel resonance, even if it doesn't make rational sense.

Occasionally, people struggle with working on a Death Wish even after muscle testing confirms that a Death Wish Pattern is present. When they speak the words, "A part of me wants to die," they say that the words don't resonate with them. In this circumstance, the reason is usually because the Death Wish is unconscious. When a Death Wish is unconscious, it may play out in (1) the physical realm, at which point we may have no conscious awareness of it until we find ourselves very sick. (In this case, it is important to note that there well may be other contributing causes for the disease state that should always be checked out with a medical doctor.) Or, (2) in our relationship with life. One extreme example of this is a client who came in with a Death Wish that he said did not resonate with him at all. Upon questioning, it turned out that he had had *thirteen* car accidents, many of them serious.

Sometimes the belief, "I want to die," actually means, "I want to experience dying." This is the case if the client is in a story where they died in another lifetime or in an imagined story, and the death was so traumatic that part of them in the story left the body before they had died so that they wouldn't have to experience the physical or emotional pain associated with the death. (Remember Sylvia in Chapter 5, who got beheaded.) This is similar to reports by people who "die" on an operating table and are brought back. They report that during the "death," they hovered above the operating table and watched what was going on as doctors frantically tried and successfully revived them. Or, it can be similar to people that have experienced extreme violence and report having witnessed the scene of violence rather than being in it. In the circumstance we are speaking of here, the body died, and there was no place to return to. It creates a need for that part to experience death to reunite and become whole again. When working with this pattern, after finding the traumatic death, the person is invited to bring all parts (including the part that had left) back into the body at the death scene and stay in the body until the death is complete. After this, the Soul can then choose to leave the body behind, leaving through the crown of the head and going to the Light. At this point, the death is complete, and in that, the Death Wish is healed.

> *When I look in the mirror and see gray hair cascading down my shoulders and the many wrinkles on my face, it feels surreal. I was never meant to live this long. In my teens, my goal was to make it to twenty; in my twenties, few thought I'd make it to thirty. Twenty psychiatric hospitalizations, five suicide attempts, heroin, crack, and alcohol addiction, and financial poverty are etched on my face. It's a miracle I am still here at all, alive and kicking, never mind sometimes thriving.*

A middle-aged woman thinking longingly of death, the axe blade still half-sunk in me, hemorrhaging something essential and unseen by the naked eye, I entered my first LCT session with little hope. "I really can't take it anymore," I confessed. "I want to die if the pain doesn't stop." Tears broke out of me like a thunderclap. I cupped my hands over my face and sobbed. When I looked up with red, glassy eyes, the paradoxical details of my life surfaced.

My highest intention was a "death wish," which didn't surprise me, given that I had begun contemplating suicide at fifteen. Per Andy's instructions, I located where I held the wish to die in my body, closed my eyes, and opened to the sensations in my chest. After some minutes, vague pictures came to mind: a gray and yellowish haze, and a sense of falling—from a plane? The color green—grass? Then, a fire—a lit barbecue in a backyard? Finally, there was the pain from the fire and anger about dying. The best estimation I could make was that someone had pushed me from a plane, and I landed in a suburban neighborhood on a lit barbecue. As I reported this bizarre and unlikely situation, Andy periodically interjected with "Uh huh," delivered in a reassuring and encouraging voice.

I then had to reexperience all the nightmarish details of the death and stay with it until the actual death occurred. Then I looked up, saw a bright, white light and was drawn to it.

Ninety minutes later, I stepped into the bright summer day, feeling like all my stains had been scrubbed out. It felt like a putrefying elephant I had been carrying my whole life was just gone, an elephant that had been carrying my urge to die.

I couldn't believe it. So, I waited, expecting it to come back tomorrow, later in the week, or next month like a nauseatingly devoted friend who refused to leave my side. But it didn't. The urge to kill myself never returned.

More miracles followed. Two years later, I got off all of my psychi-atric medication that I had been taking in combinations of up to six or more at once for over twenty years. Then, one day my fear of people disappeared. That, too, I thought would return but never did. Feeling like I was walking on cottony clouds, I began to have friends for the first time since college. Do I believe in past lives? Does it matter? I am astonished to still be here.

—Nicki Glasser (This is an excerpt from Nicki Glasser's upcoming book, *Until I Rise Again*)

A Part of Me Wishes I Was Dead

This speaks to the experience of wanting to die. It may or may not include suicidal thoughts.

In one session, I realized that I had a death wish. It came to me that I was a widow in this place, and in my grief, a part of me wanted to die to be rejoined with my husband. After finding this story, a feeling of great calm came over me.

—Riz Jammal

Someone Who Was Supposed to Love Me Wants Me Dead; to Receive Their Love, a Part of Me Has to Die

As described previously, this statement typically applies when a parent projects onto a child something they can't own in themselves. The child buys this trait as their own, sees that the parent judges it, and then has to destroy that aspect in themselves.

A Case: I Can Breathe Again

Michael came to Life Centered Therapy because he was severely allergic to cats and wanted to attend a workshop where cats would be present. Muscle testing revealed that his cat allergy was a Death Wish. When Michael said, "Someone who is supposed to love me wants me dead," he started to have trouble breathing. When he focused on that feeling of breathing distress, a story unfolded in his mind's eye in which his mother watched him sleep; he was a mere toddler in the story. Then, his mother took a pillow, placed it over her sleeping child's face, and pressed down, trying to smother him. Michael tensed up. Thankfully, his mother couldn't go through with it and removed the pillow.

Until that session, Michael had never found this story, but it was in alignment with a feeling he had had his entire life of his mother's love eluding him. Muscle testing revealed that this was all he needed, and his cat allergy was balanced. It wasn't apparent to him how this was the cause of his allergy. I invited him to go inside to find out how they were related. He realized that he associated his mother with cats as they both are carriers of female energy, and he experienced his mother's love/affection as unpredictable, sometimes withholding and on her own terms, just like a cat. Michael was hesitant to test whether the healing worked, but he decided to try exposing himself to cats, little by little. Much to his surprise and delight, he had no reaction in the presence of cats. Michael was able to attend the training he was so looking forward to.

Fractured Boundary Pattern

If you've ever felt you are like a sieve, for example, ideas come to you and when you try to retrieve them they aren't there and they are seemingly irretrievable; or, even worse, as crazy as it sounds, that you yourself feel unfindable and irretrievable, then you know something about the felt experience of Fractured Boundaries.

INDUCTING STATEMENT • *Nothing sticks inside. / Nothing nourishes me. I leak out of myself. / I am an empty husk. / No one is home.*

Fractured Boundaries occur when a person has had such a significant trauma that it fractures the person's energy field. It is typically experienced in one of two ways: either the person literally feels like they are an empty shell, or like the nourishment they take in does not sustain them whether this is literal (food) or emotional (nurturance). Often, they feel like their healing work takes them one step forward and then one step back, having the experience that none of the treatments have lasted.

From an energetic perspective, every healing we do is held in a container of a person's energetic field. So, if the field is fractured, the energy of the healing can literally leak out, like water can leak out of a cracked glass. If this is the case, relapse occurs even after a problem seems to have been resolved.

A Case: Leaking Life Force

Susan's chief complaint was that nothing was working in her life, particularly all of her efforts to heal her anemia. No matter how much she ate, how well she ate, or whatever supplemental vitamin and mineral combinations she took, she still felt physically depleted and remained anemic.

She seemed to be having very good sessions, and at the end of each of them, she felt better and more able to face Life after resolving whatever she had worked on. Each week, however, Susan returned, saying that nothing seemed to make a lasting difference. When we did a balance on "nothing seems to make a lasting difference," even that didn't make a difference. Finally, one day, in a moment of frustration, I said, "Nothing we do sticks." This was an important, total *aha* moment. Muscle testing confirmed that this was exactly what Susan needed to work on.

Susan found a past life/imaginal story in which she experienced profound mutilation and despair. She said that she had been drawn and quartered for stealing food, and her life force was draining out of her body, yet she had not died. Once we had discovered what the true problem was, we could heal it with Light (see interventions in Chapter 14), which sealed all the holes in her energy field. She described this as being like multiple tires that had blown out and were then repaired.

At the end, Susan noticed a difference from how she felt at other sessions, though she was still skeptical about whether it would make any lasting difference. I joined her in her skepticism and suggested we have a wait-and-see attitude. Susan came in the following week smiling and said that she had a lot more physical energy and was feeling so much better. She was keeping her fingers crossed that her long-standing gastrointestinal absorption problem was also getting better. Some weeks later, after her visit with her primary care doctor, she reported that her anemia had improved.

Grudge

We all know what a grudge feels like. There is the sense that someone has done you wrong and in reaction to it you might go on strike and not respond to them, feel blinding rage, and decide they are "going to pay," or go so far away that you completely insulate yourself, making sure they will never find you. The effect of these responses to being wronged is a self-poisoning revenge that can feel "good" in the moment but is ultimately destructive.

INDUCTING STATEMENT • *My values have been violated, and I act in a way that will guarantee that they will continue to be violated.*

The Grudge Pattern occurs when you feel violated by someone's behavior and instead of addressing the situation, you react to it in a way that ensures your values will continue to be violated. Imagine a friend is not good about returning phone calls, and this bothers you. Feeling hurt, you become passive-aggressive by pulling back and sending out angry energy. Your phone then rings, you see it is your friend, and instead of picking up and being happy they called, you screen the call and don't answer. Your response to the initial insult, not answering when they *do* call, is likely to lead to you continuing to feel rejected. They may call you back even less, saying, "Whenever I try calling you back, you aren't there anyway; so I don't bother."

The key in a Grudge is to identify the value violation and where it began. Most often, the way to heal a Grudge is to go to the root cause of where the trauma was born and change your behavioral response in the story to whatever feels right. In the service of healing, anything you imagine is okay as a change of behavior. To illustrate the point, we share a story from a mentor, Dick Olney, who taught about the power of grudges in our lives.

A Case: "I Don't Give a Shit"

Dick was seeing a middle-aged man named Nick as a client. It seemed that Nick spent his life living in a very constricted and withdrawn way, constipated both figuratively and literally. When Dick explored with Nick where this behavior originated, they discovered the following scene. Nick, as a five-year-old, is sitting in the back seat of the car with his father driving. He tells his father that he needs to go to the bathroom. His dad says to Nick, "Just hold on, we're almost there." They pass two gas stations, but Nick's father doesn't stop. Finally, Nick can't contain himself anymore and soils himself, and they drive home the rest of the way in silence.

Dick then asked if Nick's dad's suggestion had been helpful, and Nick said, "No!" He said that he felt humiliated in reaction to what had happened and to his father's silence. Nick said that he was realizing that in that moment, he started to withdraw into himself and continued to do so for the rest of his life, even when Life called for something different from him.

Dick invited Nick to experience how he wasn't heard, how alienated he felt, and how he literally tried to hold it all in, to hold himself back, but to no avail. The forces of nature were more powerful than he was as a five-year-old. Dick then invited the young Nick to do something different (in Life Centered Therapy, we discover if the person in the story finds what to do differently). Dick said to young Nick that he wanted Nick to experience and imagine himself in that car. Then, on the count of three, Dick was going to invite him to do something. "One, two, three. Shit all over him [his father], experience yourself shitting all over him. Keep shitting and shitting and shitting until he's totally covered with shit." Nick did this, and then a "shit-eating grin" spread across his face. Dick reported to us that after this session, Nick's constipation, both literal and figurative, started to fully release.

A Special Application: Mutual Grudges

Mutual Grudges are a special application of the Grudge Pattern, and one of the most destructive patterns in relationships. It's active when each member of a couple has a sense that the other has violated their values, and, in reaction, becomes reactive, defensive, judgmental, and comparative, with a compulsive need to understand and to be understood. Each person becomes withdrawn and self-absorbed. While the values violation is a catalyst, it's not where the real problem lies. The problem lies in the past, most often with parents in the family of origin. There is some value violation that occurred there, and metaphorically speaking, each member of the couple unconsciously puts the head of one of the parents on the body of the partner and then tries to act out the unresolved root-cause traumatic Grudge. As you might guess, this is not a healthy situation, and many destructive things happen from this. When you are feeling particularly reactive to your partner/someone you are in relationship with, consider the possibility that you are in a Grudge structure.

A Case: Help Denied

Jim and Connie came in for couples therapy because they both felt frightened about the amount of rage Jim felt and acted out following a particular incident with Connie. When they got married, both Jim and Connie were working. When Connie became pregnant, they decided together that she would be a stay-at-home mom, and he would continue to work.

Then, right after their baby was born, Jim had a bad accident at work and had to go on workers' compensation. To make ends meet, Connie had to go back to work, leaving Jim at home to care for the baby. One day, Connie came home and saw Jim fumbling with the baby's diaper, and said, in a way that she meant to be playful, "What a stupid way to be doing that!" At this, Jim hauled off and slugged her. Both came to therapy very frightened—he, for the rage that felt out of control, and she for being hit by a man who had never displayed such behavior before.

Connie's Story

Connie was the first person to share. The whole situation of having to go back to work was very difficult for her. She had really wanted to be a stay-at-home mom and take care of their baby, and it felt like Life was being a little bit unfair that Jim had had the accident and she had to work. But she was a pragmatist and did what needed to be done.

She had seen Jim struggling with the diapers before and wanted to help, but he said that he wanted to do it himself. This was very frustrating because it seemed easier for her to do, and she really wanted to care for their baby. But he was adamant and was doing a good-enough job, so she decided to let it be. She had intended to be playful when she said that it was a stupid way to do the diapers, yet she owned that maybe some of her frustration may have leaked through. Whether her frustration leaked through or not, nothing warranted his hitting her.

I asked Connie how the whole thing ought to have gone if it went exactly the way she wanted. She had wished Jim had asked her what this unexpected way of living was like for her, as opposed to just being preoccupied with what it was like for him. As she was thinking about it, she said that she truly wished that they had talked about what it was like for both of them and how life was going to be different, as opposed to just pushing through. Finally, she said that she wished he could have accepted her offer of help when she clearly was more competent at changing diapers than he was, and could have acknowledged this with a sense of appreciation.

Jim, who had been listening intently, said that he could give her exactly what she wanted in the way that she wanted it. He initiated a conversation with her in the office where he asked her what it was like for her to have to go back to work when they had had an agreement that she was going to be able to stay home and be with the baby. Just asking this made her almost tear up. She indicated that she didn't want to answer the question right away, but that she was very grateful for it and wanted to just hear what more he had to say. He then said that he was so sorry that he let his pride get in the way of being able to accept her help, and that he would do better in the future. She said that this was exactly what she wanted.

Jim's Story

Then it was Jim's turn to share and work. While he could choose to work on any incident he wanted to, he decided to share about the same experience. He described it in essentially the same way Connie did. He'd been trying his best to do the diapers because, even though he felt clumsy, he wanted to do his part for them, both as a couple and as a family. I asked Jim how he would have liked the incident to have gone if it had happened in the best way possible. Jim said that all he wanted Connie to say was that she could see how difficult this was for him, that it wasn't something he was used to doing, and that she appreciated that he was doing the very best he could. I asked her if she would do this, and she said that of course she would. She replayed the scene exactly as he wished. He said it was perfect. While doing this seemed to help some, Jim still clearly appeared to be agitated.

Connie's Family of Origin

I then invited Connie to go into the current incident and notice what sensation she was feeling in the body when she fully allowed her sense of injustice, her sense that her spouse wasn't interested in her feelings, and her experience of feeling rejected when she offered help. As she was scanning her body, she said that she was feeling nauseous to the point of almost wanting to vomit and that both her chest and her throat were tightening.

I then asked Connie to let go of the current situation so that we could find out what she was bringing to it and to bring all of her attention to the sensations and let them share. Connie started to gently cry. "I'm a little girl, maybe seven or eight, and I'm with my mother as she's putting drapes on the windows. I can see that there's a better way to do it than the way she is doing it. I say to her, 'Mommy let me help you; I know a better way to do this.' And you know what she said to me? She said, 'Just go outside and play with your friends."' Then, continuing to cry, Connie said, "I just started to cry and ran off to my room. I didn't want to go outside and play with my 'silly' friends. I wanted to take care of Mom, and she wouldn't let me. And when I ran off to my room crying, she didn't even come to comfort me or see why I was so upset. She just left me all alone crying."

I gently asked Connie how the scene ought to have gone. Connie said, "She should've let me help her. I told her that I saw a better way. All she had to do was ask me." At this point, Connie, being fully immersed in the memory, broke down crying again.

I then invited Jim to stand in as Connie's mom. He said to Connie, "I'm so sorry I didn't accept your offer of help. And that instead all I did was push you away. I am so, so, sorry." At this point, Connie melted into Jim's arms, and he hugged her very firmly and very gently.

Jim's Family of Origin

I asked Jim to take his attention away from the current situation and to allow the experience of feeling stupid and unappreciated in the eyes of someone whose acceptance was important to him. Just as he did this, his throat started to tighten up. Dropping into "Tight Throat," Jim started to cry. "I'm an eight-year-old boy, and I'm trying to help my father on a job. I am trying to shovel the gravel, but the shovel is too big for me, and I am having such a hard time. I look up, and I see my father whispering to another man, 'Look at my stupid kid, he can't even shovel the gravel right.'"

Jim said that all he wanted was for his father to acknowledge that he was trying to help and doing the best he could, and that he appreciated his effort. I asked Connie if she was willing to reenact the scene as Jim's father the way it ought to have been. Showing Jim the depth and level of understanding that he longed for, Connie, as the father, embraced him and told him exactly what he needed to hear. Jim dissolved in tears. When she was done, holding him through his sobs, Connie turned to me and said that for all the time they were married, she had never seen him cry.

Working with Mutual Grudges

In general, the way to work with Mutual Grudges is to have each partner take turns describing a scene that didn't work between them. It does not have to be the same scene. Working one person at a time, we have each of them find the sensation associated with the destructive interaction, become the sensation from the inside out, and let it share what the experience was like. It's not relevant if the listening partner, partner number two, experienced the scene in a profoundly different way.

The first partner is then asked to experience the scene exactly the way it ought to have been—to feel and embody it. Then, we ask the listening partner to reenact the scene exactly the way the first partner wanted it to be (the caveat being that they never have to do it outside of this exercise) so that the first partner can see it is possible. We keep reenacting the scene until the first partner says that they got exactly what they desired. When that is complete, we shift to the second partner and repeat the same exercise for a scene they feel didn't work between them, reenacting it until they feel satisfied.

When this is complete, we move to where the Grudge originated, finding that place/time through muscle testing. We have partner number one focus and become the sensation again and share the original story. After finding the story, the person drops inside and determines exactly how they would have wanted the story to be. The second partner now stands in for the violating person in the story and enacts it exactly how their partner wanted it to be. When this is done to the first partner's satisfaction, the first partner is complete, and we move to the second partner to repeat the whole process. After the second partner completes the same process for their story, the two can discuss what they've learned and what it was like for them if any of that feels useful.

Neglect Pattern

We've all had the experience at one time or another of feeling "Where are you when I need you? You promised you'd be here with me, but you're nowhere to be found." A feeling of desperation can ensue from this sense of abandonment. In reaction, you may say to yourself, *I'll never put myself in this position again, and I'll never let myself need anybody*, yet underneath, there's a clinging and a holding-on. We may feel the craving and neediness, the pulling away and becoming an island, or the limiting of desire and overresponsibility. No matter which of these becomes predominant, Neglect will keep us from truly being able to know our own needs, be intimate with another, and be autonomous. Do any of these variations of Neglect resonate with you in your life?

INDUCTING STATEMENT • *When I really needed you as though my life depended on it, you were not there for me.*

A Neglect Pattern occurs when a person perceived that they needed someone for their actual survival (emotionally or physically), and that person was not there for them. There is a sense of abandonment. It can be severely traumatic because the experience is often one in which the person literally perceives their life as being threatened; the baby screaming for its mother may believe that they will die if the mother does not show up. Frequently, when this pattern is operative, the person has internalized negative parental messages.

Neglect traumas are different from all other traumas in that they are based on acts of *omission*, while other traumas are based on acts of *commission*. Because neglect is an act of omission, people don't always initially resonate with the pattern in their lives.

Neglect plays out situationally with something like the person saying, "You traumatized me," and the other person responds, "What are you talking about? I didn't do anything." The traumatized person then says, "That is exactly the point. You didn't do anything."

There are many variations on how Neglect patterns present. The classic example would be depression with a strong sense of hopelessness and neediness, and/or a blocking of depression by being self-reliant and taking action in the world while denying having any needs at all.

A Case: In Your Arms

Ava, a twenty-five-year-old woman, had been coming to therapy for about a year when her father died. Prior to this session, she had just returned from a trip to her parents' home to go to his memorial service. She was feeling very anxious when she returned to Boston, and she wasn't exactly clear why she was feeling even more afraid and more wistful about the past than she had been. Muscle testing indicated that what she most needed to work on was a Neglect trauma that originated in her lifetime between the ages of birth to five. Something about this trauma was making the difficult loss of her father even worse.

When Ava scanned her body to notice what sensations were associated with neglect, she felt a deep hollowness and pressure in her chest that felt to her like severe emotional pain.

Becoming "Hollowness and Pressure in Chest," she reported, "I'm see- ing myself as a toddler, an older infant. I'm at the edge of my playpen, and my arms are up. I am so badly wanting to be picked up. I see my dad, and he walks past me. He doesn't or can't pick me up." Ava began to cry, "I'm in agony. I'm feeling an intense desire to be held. It's so painful to not be picked up. And I'm feeling so scared. I'm starting to have a temper tantrum. I so want to be noticed, and it's so frustrating. It seems like he's absent so much. I just want his attention. I miss him affirming me that I'm the one he most loves. Since he's died, I feel like I will never be picked up again. This may sound crazy, but I believe now that he's died, he will forget about me. He's in the spirit world, and it's so good there. Why would he care about me anymore? I'm afraid of being forgotten. At least when he was alive, I had a hope that he would not forget about me. I didn't realize how special it is to be so loved—so loved the way parents love you."

As Ava was saying the end of this, she had the sense that a golden Light was coming down from the heavens and surrounding her in a way that seems like an egg. Something about this seemed very healing to her even though she had no particular associations to it. She could only say that the hollowness was filling in, the pressure was releasing, and along with it, the deepest of the emotional pain.

This session is very instructive about the seeming insignificance of a moment. Often, parents are unable to pick up their child when the child calls. Why would this be such a significant moment for Ava? Freud suggests an answer to this question in a term he coined *screen memory*, which he described in an 1899 paper by the same name. He said that seemingly bland memories of early childhood are hooked to more significant, less innocent occurrences that somehow get captured by the relatively harmless scene.

Wounded Pattern

If you have a sense of overresponsibility in your life with an underlying sense of guilt that you can't quite explain, or you find yourself sabotaging advancement into positions of power because there seems to be a vague underlying fear of not being able to handle the responsibility, you may have to work with a Wounded Pattern. It can even show up as consistently denying your own needs or desires out of guilt or unworthiness. Any of this resonate?

INDUCTING STATEMENT • *I have betrayed.*

With a Wounded Pattern, a person perceives that they have broken a commitment and suffers guilt or shame at their failure to fulfill their responsibility. The theme of betrayal can occur in any role: mother, father, teacher, political leader, healer, friend, and so forth. Living life through the lens of a Wounded Pattern can cause people to be overly responsible in their lives because of the guilt about letting others down in the past. Or, they may fear taking responsibility because they anticipate letting others down. Often, a client will come in saying that whenever they get near a position of authority and power, they unconsciously sabotage themselves.

An often-seen story is when the person was a spiritual leader, experiencing that they have made a sacred covenant with God/Source to lead their people to the "promised land," whatever the particulars of that may be. In the story, the person breaks the covenant by betraying the community (e.g., running away when threatened by outside forces); betraying Source (e.g., losing faith); or betraying themselves (e.g., breaking a vow of celibacy). In all stories of betrayal, but particularly in these types, people often have the experience of having difficulty finding a sense of agency in their lives and accessing their power because they have an unconscious fear of abusing it.

A Case: Wounded Pride and Judgment

Charlie is a fifty-five-year-old consultant and teacher with a ruddy, outdoorsy look and a firm and gentle manner. He came to treatment for several reasons: (1) He had difficulty making enough money even though he felt that he ought to be successful; (2) He had ongoing, low-grade anxiety; and (3) He had a very difficult relationship with his daughter who seemed to be getting into deeper and deeper trouble despite his best efforts to help her. Although he felt capable of intimate relationships in general, he felt he was unable to have one with his daughter. He felt self-conscious when he interacted with her and always felt as if he was walking on eggshells.

Muscle testing revealed that none of these were his intention; instead, it turned out that his intention was a Wounded Pattern that originated in a karmic past life/the imaginal realms. Charlie then made the inducting statement, "I betrayed a sacred trust." Muscle testing affirmed a particularly strong yes. Tears came, and Charlie said, "I have a terrible pain in my heart." He said that he felt he had betrayed his daughter because when he and his wife had divorced, she took the daughter away, and Charlie felt that he had abandoned her. He had promised her he would protect her no matter what, and he felt that he had broken this covenant.

While this was true, muscle testing revealed that this was not where the pattern had originated. This was not surprising because originally, the muscle testing had indicated that the root cause was in a karmic past life/imaginal realm. I asked Charlie to really focus on the pain in his heart, and

I said, "Pain in the Heart, where are you originating? What's happening? Who are you? Where are you?" Charlie responded, "I am a priest walking away in disgust from the parish where I ministered. They are so caught up in money and greed, and nothing I do can get through to them. Instead of asking God for help, I see myself walking away from the town, feeling like a total failure. I pull out a knife and impulsively thrust it into my heart." Though he was deeply in the story, he stopped himself and said, "I've always had such judgment about people who committed suicide. Now I know why. And I can see why I've had such issues around greed and how this has stopped me from feeling free about making money." Charlie went on to share, "I have abandoned those who are entrusted to my care. I am disgusted with them and myself. I was not responsible enough."

I then invited Charlie to come back fully in his body in that lifetime and to let himself fully die and go to *Bardo*, the time between lives. We discovered that the primary person that Charlie had betrayed was himself as well as betraying his parishioners, and, as he talked to his Soul, it told him that this was his opportunity to truly crack open his heart. Charlie realized as he opened his heart that this would likely profoundly affect his relationship with his daughter because he could be more lovingly present with her, instead of being caught up in his own angst about his helplessness, which had caused his suicide so many lifetimes ago. As he realized this his tears of suffering shifted into tears of joy, and where there was a gaping, painful wound, he now reported a golden, glowing light.

Double-Bind Pattern

Have you ever felt crazy because it feels like what someone says and what they do are not in alignment, but you can't quite put your finger on the issue, and worse yet, you don't feel capable of addressing it with them? If you have a sense of what we are talking about here, you may be experiencing a Double Bind.

INDUCTING STATEMENT • *If I get what I want, something even* *worse will happen than if I don't get what I want, and my reality about this will be denied.*

The concept of double-binds was introduced by one of the most brilliant thinkers of the twentieth century, the systems theorist Gregory Bateson. A Double-Bind Pattern exists when a person experiences that they are doomed, regardless of what option they take: "Damned if I do, and damned if I don't." It typically presents with clients feeling crazy or paralyzed in the context of getting what they want in life. They sense that if they get what they want, something even worse will happen than if they don't get their desires met at all.

An example of this might be a child who wants affection from their parent and asks for a hug. When the parent holds out their arms, the child runs forward but then feels their parent stiffen. The child may take the stiffening to mean that the parent doesn't love them or is ambivalent about the love. The child, responding to the stiffening, backs away. The parent, perhaps not recognizing and certainly not owning the part they played in the child's reaction asks, "What's the matter? Don't you want a hug?" or, even worse, "Don't you love me?"

If the child could speak, and the power dynamic was even, the child might say something like, "It's not me that seems not to want to hug; it's you. You held out your arms, and then, when I ran into them, you stiffened while we hugged. This makes me believe that what you say you want and what you want on a deeper level are not the same. And while I'm afraid this has something to do with me, I'm much surer it has something to do with you. I really wish you would look at yourself and see what's going on because it's so painful to me."

The child believed that the hug would let him feel loved, and this is not the case. The way to understand what really happened from the child's perspective is: "My parent is ambivalent in their love for me," which is the least acceptable way to make sense of it for the child. In order to keep the possibility alive of receiving the love, the child has two choices. First, he can choose to doubt his perception that the parent recoiled and convince himself that he was just imagining it. Or second, he can say that it is his fault that the parent might be ambivalent. This allows him to continue to believe that the parent is a person from whom he *can* receive love, and that if he acts differently, he will receive it. This second choice also supports the child blaming himself when he is not to blame at all. Unfortunately, the problem must be solved by the parent and not the child.

When this child grows up, when their partner expresses ambivalence, they will react like they did as the child, either doubting themselves or doing whatever it takes to get their partner to be able to express their love for them unambivalently.

A very simple way of understanding the structure of a Double-Bind Pattern is:

- If I don't get A → then B (something negative)
- If I do get A → then C (C is unconscious and even worse than B)

A variation on this theme is:

- In order to survive/thrive → I need something.
- It is impossible to get what I need.

A Case: Crazy-Making Dissonance

Because we feel this is a complex concept to understand, we just present a clear scenario as an example instead of using a real case.

Suppose your new boss says, "I want you to know that I value openness and honesty, and I'd like you all to share with me any problems or concerns that you have." Then one of your well-respected colleagues steps forward and shares his ideas. That colleague, who up until now has been the golden boy in the department, starts to be assigned less-than-choice projects, even though there seems no apparent reason for this. It is so subtle that no one, including you, is exactly aware of what is going on, yet there is an almost unnamable, insidious feeling that something is wrong. People then have a pervasive sense of being on guard, but there is nothing to pin it on, and it doesn't feel safe to talk about. As a result, what happens is that people stop talking to the new boss in the way he has requested, and they never talk to each other about it.

Sometime later in a staff meeting, the boss says he feels disappointed because, even though he has asked for candid feedback for quite some time, no one has spoken up. Each person in the department independently has a sense of trepidation about being honest with the boss, but no one can seem to remember what it was born of or talks about it. Therefore, their internal response is that they have fallen short of their boss's request, and as a result, they begin to believe that they have done something wrong. They feel sort of paralyzed and crazy. What never gets talked about because the boss is the boss is the perception that the boss "talks the talk but doesn't walk the walk," and the impact of that on the department.

This fits the Double-Bind Pattern structure. You, as the employee, might really want to be able to talk to your boss about your concerns, and if you are not able to do so, you might feel a kind of disenchantment. Yet, you have an unconscious fear that if you do talk with your boss, something even worse than disenchantment will arise, that you will be powerless and dead-ended. We can also see the two different levels of communication. Verbally, your boss says, "Come and talk with me." Yet through his actions, you perceive he is saying the exact opposite. Nonetheless, you also perceive that it is impossible to talk about the situation because if you did, you sense that, at best, your boss would deny anything you bring up and resent you, which could have adverse implications. At worst, he could make your life miserable. All of this would be subtle enough that you would not be able to step back and perceive what was going on. Instead, you might feel that something is terribly wrong with the situation, and you might even feel that there was something very wrong with you.

Conclusion

We have shared a great deal of information with you here and many client experiences. We chose cases that clearly, directly, and concisely exemplified the pattern we were trying to illustrate. While no two sessions look alike, we do see cases all the time that look like these. Sometimes, resolution of symptoms occurs almost immediately. It is almost like each session is a gift that you can tie a bow around and put away.

Other times, it truly is like an archaeological dig (see Appendix, Blocked Patterns, Muriel), with small discoveries that keep adding to the development of an overarching narrative that, if we stay with the metaphor, begins to bring us to an understanding of the entire development and civilization of one's Soul.

Perhaps the most powerful reason to explore these patterns is the amount of transformation you can experience in a very short period. Many seemingly disparate problems, which may appear to have nothing to do with each other, can transform when we find the higher order theme in which they are all enfolded.

As we said earlier, you may find that certain themes seem more operative to you than others. In terms of your healing journey, we recommend that you begin with those and see what your body has to share with you about what *your* story is.

CHAPTER 9

Triple-Center Patterns in the Nonmaterial Realms: What You Can't See Can Hurt You

W e're about to enter a topic about which many of you may say, "Thank God!" Others may say, "You've got to be kidding!" or "That sounds crazy!" Still, others may say, "I've never thought about the question, and it's never really mattered to me." At the outset, what we would like to emphasize most is that whether you believe the following stories are literally true, metaphorically true, or can't possibly be true doesn't really matter in the context we are sharing here. *What we and our clients most care about is how useful the work is.* If, for example, when you have tinnitus and our diagnostic system suggests that the symptom of tinnitus and a story of an extraterrestrial implant are exactly the same, and you find the story and transform it, with a cessation of your tinnitus, you are not likely to care so much one way or the other if this story is literally true or not. And if you do, much has been written about both sides of the question.

We now turn to healing suffering that originates in trauma in what we call the nonmaterial realms. These realms include such phenomena that we refer to as an Entity, Ghost, Curse, Superimposition (energies that are bigger than us, that take us over), and Extraterrestrial. Included are the ideas of gods and goddesses, guides, and angels that can be both victims of these traumas and possible aids in healing them. These concepts are controversial and not held in mutually agreed-upon reality in Western culture because they are not perceived by the five senses, are not experienced by everyone, and cannot be documented in a satisfactorily quantifiable way for Western science to acknowledge.

As we have said earlier, even though the traumas themselves may not be experienced through the five senses, invariably, the consequences of them are. If, for example, a person wants to put a curse on you that you will have back pain, which is the trauma, and intends to amplify the power of the curse by sticking a pin into the back of a voodoo doll, while you certainly won't experience the pin literally going into your back, you might (or might not) experience pain in your back.

As would be true with any topic that has generated such controversy, our invitation is to be open to this material with skepticism and curiosity in healthy balance, and further to open to how much this material resonates with your own deepest subjective experience, even if it might not seem so rational to your conscious Western mind. In our experience, these concepts aren't considered in standard mental-health practice, and if a client brings up an experience of this type, it is either deemed irrelevant, dismissed, or pathologized (regarded as psychologically abnormal or unhealthy). Our intention here is to describe the usefulness of opening to these concepts.

This usefulness demonstrates itself in many ways. On the simplest level, it has helped honor the personal reality of people who have been concerned that they would be unacknowledged or worse, stigmatized, should they speak and live their truth. Second, it has helped give language to people who were having experiences that they couldn't account for in any familiar way. They had a knowing that they were having a problem without being able to name what the problem was.

Finally, when we open to the nonmaterial realms, it follows that we consider resources for healing that civilizations of people have relied on for time eternal for comfort and healing—prayer in its many forms. This includes opening to God/Life/Source, whatever the understanding of this is for you. You will notice that we capitalize the word Light in many places in this chapter; when we do this, we are referring to one of the faces of the Divine. God/Life/Source is bigger and more powerful than any type of demonic energy or any of the things we are most afraid to experience. As long as we remember this, it really doesn't make that much difference whether we are dealing with a trauma in which a client experiences that they have been taken over by a dark energy or a trauma, in which a client feels that a parent has yelled at them, and they couldn't handle it.

What is most important to reiterate is this: *what typically is least important here is the literal truth of these phenomena.* Whether we make sense of these patterns as being literally true or a metaphor for internal experience is not significant for healing to occur. What is typically very important is the theme that is associated with the pattern. Anything that takes you over can qualify as a Superimposition whether it's a dark energy, an emotion, an idea, an addiction, or an obsession.

Finally, the very same experience can map in profoundly different ways (the diagnostic decision tree used in our protocol can lead you to different places and different names for the experience) depending on how you undergo the experience. Let's suppose that you became part of a cult and ultimately experienced this as a very traumatic life event. One client may work on this trauma directly. A second client may experience the trauma as an Extraterrestrial implant. That would be a clue that it felt like something literally had been put inside them and was running their life, or even that they were being experimented on. A third client might experience it as a Superimposition, having felt like something much larger than them had taken them over and was holding them down. A fourth client might experience the trauma as a Ghost and feel haunted by the experience. The beauty of the diagnostic is that it will reveal a clue to the person's inner subjective experience that may be profoundly useful for them in healing.

Now let's look at the nonmaterial realm patterns.

Entity

An Entity, in our framework, is a being with animal-like qualities that can attach to a person and have a draining effect. Again, as we pointed out before, as in all patterns, *the key is the theme* of the pattern and not necessarily the narrative content. For example, while an Entity may narratively be like a little, nonhuman energetic being, it may also be something like your job. Let's suppose that you have some kind of trauma around your work, and you're not exactly clear about what it is, and it comes out in muscle testing that the trauma equals an Entity. When you drop into the sensation and become it, you might come to the realization that your job is like a parasite that is sucking you dry.

A Case: Sucking the Life Out of Me

Stephanie called with acute physical symptoms that needed attention. She had a history of asthma, but after ten years of drug therapy that had ended five years earlier, she was symptom free. Then, seemingly out of nowhere, she began to experience severe asthmatic symptoms again. Stephanie had cleaned out her basement several days before the symptoms returned, and she believed that the dust/mold exposure in the basement was the likely cause of her relapse. Stephanie called her primary care physician who started her on her former asthma treatment regime for a month's duration. In her previous experience with this drug combination, it had taken two to four weeks for its effects to really kick in.

At a Life Centered Therapy session Stephanie had the day after she started the medication, she discovered through muscle testing that the asthma symptoms were the equivalent of an Entity. Stephanie made the inducting statement of the Entity pattern: "Something has attached itself to me and is draining my energy." Open to aligning with it, Stephanie became aware that the physical sensations of chest constriction and shortness of breath were becoming more pronounced.

By fully focusing on the constriction and shortness of breath, she dropped her consciousness into the part of her that was experiencing the Entity and reported the following story: "There is a group of small creatures with oblong bodies and elongated arms. There is a dark, dungeon-like scene with a cauldron, and there is a wizard-like being who collapses as light is brought to him. Oh, and there is a Pegasus creature that is flying out of the cauldron."

Muscle testing indicated that the entities had attached to her during the basement cleaning, and that Stephanie was somehow vulnerable to their intrusion in a way that could be corrected by surrounding herself in Source Light. (We will talk about this and other interventions in Chapter 14.) While it may or may not be literally true that these little creatures were attached to her, what is certainly true is that Stephanie subjectively experienced a resolving of her symptoms and the anxiety that accompanied them when they dissolved.

Stephanie's literal experience was that the entities were controlled by the wizard, and when the wizard died, they did, too. She realized that the wizard represented men in her life who had undermined her rather than supported her—they never made her life *magical*. Stephanie also realized that her life choices were suffocating her, and Stephanie needed to step out and enjoy Life more, breathe more vitality into her life, and not worry about mundane responsibilities like cleaning the basement.

Upon leaving that therapy session, Stephanie reported that her chest felt clear and her breathing was easy. She felt she no longer needed the meds but made an appointment with her doctor just to be sure. The doctor listened to her lungs and concurred that the medication was no longer necessary. Stephanie has not had a problem since, even when cleaning her basement.

Ghost

Ghosts are energies that were, at one time, human beings. They become problematic for people when they attach themselves to them and start draining their energy or having some other negative impact. The complexity when dealing with a Ghost Pattern is that it can sometimes be difficult to differentiate whether the symptoms a person is experiencing are the person's in relationship to the ghost or the ghost's itself. Perhaps the most problematic Ghost stories, which are quite unusual, are stories in which the ghost has taken over the person, and the person is experiencing life through the ghost. Often, these people come in feeling like zombies because they have identified with the dead. Once again, we wish to reiterate that a key with a Ghost Pattern is a theme. If somebody is haunting you, metaphorically speaking, muscle testing could diagnose a Ghost. The same diagnosis can happen if someone you care about "ghosted you" (suddenly disappears, loses contact with you). Other times, people experience an energy that was once a part of another human being. It's all about theme.

People can develop codependent relationships with ghosts, making it difficult and frightening to let them go. They may also hold onto a ghost because they themselves have not completed a grieving process. A fascinating example of an entirely different way of having a "ghost" is described in the book, *A Change of Heart*, by Claire Sylvia. After Claire had a heart transplant, she started drinking, wanting to smoke, and acting very differently. She discovered that the way she was acting exactly replicated the way of being of the man whose heart she had received.

Or, as in a case we are about to discuss, ghosts can attach themselves because they have not found their way to Source and are trying to hold on to their lives as they knew it. This may be particularly relevant for ghosts that people pick up in places often associated with death, such as cemeteries, battlefields, or hospitals. This can also be important if a person lives in a home where someone had a traumatic death.

Ghosts can come from motivations that are benevolent and/or malevolent. They can come to someone they have loved or can attach randomly. We will illustrate some of these possibilities.

A Case: Hanging On

We will now turn to two stories in which each client had the same symptom—a physical symptom described as "like having a noose around my neck." The feeling made each person so uncomfortable that they literally could not wear turtleneck sweaters, scarves, or anything tight around their necks. Each woman also described depressive symptoms.

In the first case, Lulu discovered that the noose-like quality was the ghost of her father who had hanged himself. It became clear when she dropped into body sensation that he had not been ready to leave her, nor had she been ready to let him go. During the session, Lulu went through a final deep-mourning process for her father and was able to finally let him go after more than two decades. Lulu experienced her father going to the Light of Source. Lulu's depressive symptoms, including elements of unfinished mourning, her father's depressive structure, and the ambivalence that had characterized their relationship, all released. Lulu's depression significantly lightened, and her physical neck symptom never returned.

A Case: Mother Love

The second client, Bridget, had had a difficult several years. Diagnosed with a malignancy in her neck, she had required extensive surgery to ensure her best chance for a full recovery. In addition to the introspection that a serious diagnosis like this tends to invite, Bridget was dealing with a very unusual and agitating symptom *after* the surgery which plagued her every waking hour. She was experiencing a sensation that she described as "having a noose tied around my neck." Bridget said it was "maddening." Each night, she would tear off her clothes, hoping that that would bring relief.

Bridget was frustrated because her surgeon told her repeatedly that nothing about the surgery could account for this problem. Even though she professed to be grateful that she had been healthy since the surgery, and even though she "protested" that she ought to feel wonderful about how things were working out, Bridget was not happy. Her unhappiness bordered on depression. This didn't make sense to her, and she also felt guilty for her lack of gratitude.

When Joni did a diagnostic with Bridget, they found that a Ghost Pattern accounted for both her depression and her strange neck sensation. Bridget reported, "This makes total sense to me because last week I had a very strange idea. It came to me that this uncomfortable sensation was caused by a ghost I picked up during surgery. This seemed so outrageous to me that I dismissed it."

As Bridget began to focus on the noose-like feeling in her neck, she became aware of a community of little ghost children who were saying that they wanted their mommies, that she was like their mommies, and that they wanted to stay with her.

In that moment, Bridget realized that the feeling was focused in her neck because it was the place of her greatest vulnerability. She felt that these ghost children were hanging onto her neck for dear life. And if these ghosts were real, it made sense that they would be drawn to her because when she had entered surgery, she was thinking about her children and asking God to keep her well so she could be there for them as they grew up.

Bridget further realized that much of her depression stemmed from her lack of consideration of herself. She was so worried about being there for her children that she had doubled down on mothering, and she spent extraordinarily little time or energy on caring for herself, even with the wake-up call of the diagnosis and surgery. At this time, it became apparent how the physical symptom, the ghosts, and unhappiness/depression were all really one difficulty. Her susceptibility to the ghosts and her inability to let go of them, and her blindness to taking care of her own needs, mirrored each other.

This awareness was the necessary step to be able to release the ghosts. Bridget was then able to explain with empathy to the ghost children that she understood that they missed their mommies, but that they had to go. She then invited the ghosts' energies to return to Source by telling them they could go to a place where they could be even happier. She reported: "During the story, I could feel the children's longing, pain, and agitation; and when they left, I felt a peaceful and calm quietness."

Later, Bridget was able to constructively determine ways to care for herself while still being available to her children. She realized that she could actually be more attentive to them if she was more attentive to her own needs.

Several years have passed since this session. The sensation that was so agitating to Bridget has never recurred. She has accepted the need to listen to the ongoing call of self-care and to provide the nourishment she requires to thrive.

My dad comes from an extremely abusive family. Imagine your worst nightmare, and multiply it by three. He was a victim of sexual, physical, and verbal abuse. People didn't want to believe him because the things were too horrible to bear. In short, my grand father was a monster of a man. When my dad turned eighteen, he decided to no longer have a relationship with his father. I was kept away from my grandfather my whole life. My grandfather died when I was fourteen. When my dad got the news, he hung up the phone and said, "I've been waiting my whole life for this day." Then, he went back to mowing the lawn.

Years later, my husband and I moved into my childhood home in New Hampshire. I woke up in the middle of the night with a feeling that someone was in my house. The feeling washed through me from head to toe—a wave of awareness that my husband and I were not alone. Without disturbing my husband, I walked out of the bedroom to investigate. I found my grandfather sitting six or seven feet away from me in the corner. He was hunched over, and he looked up at me. A surge of fear shocked my senses. I knew who it was, and I knew what he did. He looked solid—as if he were still alive—but I knew he was dead. I didn't know what I was deal-ing with; was this a demonic spirit or something else? I did NOT want to interact—I felt like that would be playing with fire. Anger bordering on rage fueled me to speak: "Get out!" He vanished the moment the words escaped my lips.

But he kept coming back to me. It was awful. I was exhausted and becoming increasingly anxious that he'd show up, which he did. Eventually, I asked, "What do you want from me?"

My grandfather answered, "I want to confess to you. I'm in Bardo —in the in-between. I'm stuck. I'm so afraid to move on because I'm afraid of what's on the other side for me because I did some really horrible things."

He then proceeded to show me the things he did—I could see them like a movie in my mind as if they were my own memories. It was horrible. I saw all of the abuse inflicted on my grandmother, on my dad, and on my six aunts and uncles when they were children.

I told my dad this story later, including the story of one particu-larly upsetting scene I'd witnessed in which the children were all seated at the dinner table with my grandfather when my grand-father rose and beat my grandmother unconscious. Then my dad, who was around age ten at the time, got up and ran to the neigh-bor's house to tell them to call the police—that was his job in the family. I could see him running through the trees in the darkness, and hear the crisp fall leaves crunching under his frantic pace.

When I finished telling the story, my dad said, "Where was every-one sitting at the table in that story?"

"Why?" I asked.

"I want you to confirm for me where everyone sat because I want to confirm that it's really my dad coming through to you."

I traced the oval table in the air for him and pointed to each of my aunts and uncles in turn to confirm.

My dad erupted. "I don't want him in the f***ing house!" He was so angry because he didn't want his father to affect me—not during his life and certainly not after it. He told me not to have anything to do with him—to stay away.

But what I discovered to be true for me is that if you have these abilities to interact with people who have passed, you cannot pick and choose who you want to help. It's in your soul contract to help everyone who comes to you and especially when they come to you asking for help and forgiveness. But my dad had said no.

After my session, I told my dad that I knew he didn't want me to talk with my grandfather, but that maybe he should then talk with him and finish it. In an LCT session, my dad was able to communicate with his father, who then moved on and away from us. It helped my dad to make peace with his past and move on, having healed a big part of himself. Since that day, neither one of us has seen or felt my grandfather's presence.

—Erica Barnes

Curse

Curses are about the power of malevolent intention. When beings desire, feel, and intend maliciousness toward another being, trauma can result.

As a trauma structure, a person can be the one who curses, is cursed, or both. Curses come in two types—personal or archetypal. When a curse is personal, it is directed at a person as retribution. When it's archetypal, the curse isn't personal. Rather, it's about what the person or group represents. An Archetypal Curse Pattern can be about race, ethnicity, nationality, gender, or class, to name a few examples. If an archetypal curse is directed at a particular person, then that person is invariably famous like a politician, an athlete, or an entertainer. In that case, the person inflicting the curse doesn't know the celebrity personally. Rather, the curse is cast because of something like racism or sexism.

Curses can occur in this dimension or in other dimensions. A dimension is simply a level of consciousness or existence. Our dimension that we experience every day is our life here on Earth as we know it. Other dimensions are other imagined or unseen worlds from our perspective. So, heaven and hell, for example, are other dimensions. Another example is that if you believe that it's possible that extraterrestrials could literally fly into your backyard, then from your perspective, extraterrestrials exist in our dimension. If you believe that extraterrestrials aren't "real" in that way, then they are of another dimension from your perspective. In other dimensions (unseen or imagined worlds), a typical story is about a being (often an angel) being cursed by a group who feels forsaken. When something bad happened that was out of anyone's control, often concerning the physical or spiritual survival of the group, the collective cursed the being (gods/angels). Feeling personally responsible for forces that were beyond their control, the cursed being takes on the curse projected from the group he "failed" to protect. Being weighed down by the hatred enfolded in the curse, these "Light Beings" (beings that are in unseen or imagined worlds or other dimensions who are in service to help and heal in this world, such as angels, guides, and guardians) invariably fall through the dimensions. People who present with this pattern are often plagued by feelings of guilt and over-responsibility and experience the Light Being story just like they experience a memory from their present life or an imagined story that is affecting them.

Curses can also occur on either of two types: content or process. The first type focuses on content. For example: "You will never be able to heal"; "You will never be able to have a close relationship"; and "You will never conceive and have a baby." The second and more virulent form of a Curse

Pattern focuses on foiling a person's process in trying to attain a meaningful goal. For example: "The more you try to heal, the worse you will get"; "The more intimate you try to become, the worse your relationship will be"; and "The harder you try to conceive, the worse things will get."

One woman came to Life Centered Therapy because she had been unable to conceive for seven years, even though there were no physical reasons to explain her barrenness. In the month after we balanced a process Curse Pattern she was experiencing, she got pregnant. The woman carried her baby to term and delivered a healthy child. While we have no evidence that the reason that she was able to conceive was the transformation of the Curse Pattern she experienced, the woman wholeheartedly believed that that was the case. Moreover, it's not useful to judge whether the woman was literally cursed or metaphorically cursed. What is useful is to note that healing her experience helped her to resolve and end her experience of being cursed. It is known that there are often psychological contributors that affect whether a person can conceive. There are many stories of women who tried to get pregnant for many years without success and then conceived shortly after adopting a baby, for example. The psychological component is undeniable. The woman in this example may have somehow "relaxed" about the idea of conception after we healed the Curse Pattern she experienced, and that could be what contributed to her getting pregnant.

Case One: Suffocating the Heart

Elliott had ongoing self-defeating attitudes, a sense of being blocked from really moving forward in his life, and sinus difficulties. Muscle testing indicated that a Curse was at the core of all of these problems. Elliott had some skepticism about the idea of a curse in general. But he was willing to suspend judgment and go forward with the work.

As Elliott repeated the statement, "I am cursed," and focused on his body, he said he felt like he was struck by a powerful energy. He said that he could feel anger coming at him. As his story unfolded, Elliott discovered an incident from a past life/his imagination where he had, in a position of authority, ordered the destruction of a tree that marked a person's final resting place. The person's family pleaded with him not to destroy the tree because of its sacred significance to the family, but he didn't listen. The patriarch of the family became very angry at him, and Elliott said that he could feel the man's anger stick in him like a sword. This was the beginning of Elliott's realization that things that were unseen, like emotions, could have such a strong literal impact (the curse). As he watched the tree come down, the air was filled with dust and debris, making it hard to breathe.

As the story resolved, Elliott could feel himself come to a place of compassion for both himself and the angry patriarch. Elliott found the story in its entirety, and it no longer had any charge for him because he was able to fully process it. Muscle testing revealed that Elliott had indeed found the full story of the trauma, but something else still needed to happen. Spontaneously, he said, "I'm going through a tube or tunnel. It feels so good. I feel so much joy that I want to cry. I'm safe." Experiencing that positive energy transformed the energy of the curse. The positive energy allowed him to realize "how people's feelings, while they may be materially invisible, still have real impact—as real as physical objects."

Elliott reported that he had a realization that he, like the authority in his story, had been unaware of others' feelings and incapable of developing consensus in relationships. Those things held him back. He felt confident that this newfound awareness would let him move forward in Life. He added that his sinuses were clearer as well.

Case Two: Taking on What Isn't Yours

Hillary wanted to work on her pervasive sense of guilt. "I do a lot, and it never feels like enough," she lamented. Muscle testing indicated that the underlying cause of this problem was an Archetypal Curse. Fully allowing her sense of guilt, Hillary began to feel constriction in her heart. Opening to "Heart Constriction," it shared that she was a goddess in a civilization that did not feel like it was on the Earth. She could feel a sense of absolute power and absolute helplessness at the same time. Then, while not exactly clear about what occurred next, she said, "There is some type of cataclysmic event happening." She felt a sense of responsibility to do something to help her people, but she did not have the authority in her role as a deity to do anything on the grand scale that seemed necessary to save them.

Then, she noticed a priestess in the temple that she sensed was her daughter in the story. This young woman trusted that the goddess would save them all. But the goddess was unable to save them, including her daughter, and everyone in the temple perished. As they were dying, they thought she should have saved them and they cursed her saying, "We trusted you, and you have forsaken us. You could have saved us, and you didn't; we hate you, and you deserve to suffer."

As the story unfolded, Hillary discovered a place of deep, seemingly unending grief and horror. As she allowed that feeling, she spontaneously broke into tears. The guilt and the body sensation associated with it began to subside. She then described that a golden Light began to fill her. She looked up, and in a very peaceful voice said, "I am done."

In the ensuing year, Hillary reported several major changes. As her children had reached late adolescence, she found it easier to give them space and hover less. While still supporting them, she no longer felt responsible for their choices. She felt she cared for them adequately and appropriately. She went on to then happily report that she was able to spend money on herself without feeling guilty, allowing herself many new experiences in the process.

Superimposition

Superimpositions are energies that take someone over. They "super-impose" themselves and attach when a person is vulnerable and/or has specifically asked for help without specifying from whom they are looking for it to come. They typically feed off fear or disease—physical, emotional, mental, or spiritual. Superimpositions may come from the light or the dark. A superimposition coming from the light comes with good intentions and is benevolent. A superimposition coming from the dark is coming with evil, malevolent intentions. One way to think about it is that superimpositions are agents of heaven and hell. Superimpositions from the light come in times of difficulty, with positive intentions of helping. However, if they are not released, a person can come into a codependent relationship with the energy, both then needing each other. In addition, even though a superimposition coming from the light may have good intentions, sometimes the results are not serving the intended beneficiary and need to be balanced. Superimpositions from the dark may attach under many circumstances— when a person is in a particularly vulnerable state, that is, either weakened or frightened and sick in a hospital, or walking through a cemetery at night. Or, a superimposition can attach when a person has asked for help but does not distinguish from whom he is asking for help, naively assuming the help would come from the light when, in fact, a dark superimposition, posing as a helper from the light, answers the call. Another example is when a person has a subjective experience of losing Source and is then susceptible to any kind of belonging. And finally, when a person makes a contract with the demonic realm, they invite superimpositions from the dark into their experience.

These contracts with the demonic realm may be based on the ego's fear of death—either literally of physical demise, or figuratively of emotional annihilation. This situation is particularly virulent because the dark forces can seem like they are taking control of the person's life. The person usually needs to find the part of them that was vulnerable and in need, and hence made the pact, and then renounce it. Because the pact was never legitimate in the first place (the superimposition, by definition, cannot live up to its side of the contract, and an ego cannot ultimately give away its Soul), the contract can be broken.

It is important to remember that although superimpositions from the dark, and demonic energies in particular, have a "negative" quality, they originate from Source and still serve Life. How could something that seems so evil serve Life? In order to answer this question, let's look at the story of the crucifixion of Jesus. In the story, in order for Jesus to save the world, he must have someone betray him. So Judas as betrayer is required. In the same way, all of us need a crucible in order to grow. From the perspective of Soul, everything serves Life, and good and evil do not exist. From the perspective of our humanity, it is a different story—if we see a person beating a child, we need to stop it or call the police.

It's also important to note that while working with the energy called Superimposition, that these energies can shapeshift during a session and seemingly "go into hiding" and be difficult to find. Finally, anything you experience as bigger than you that takes you over qualifies as a superimposition. While on the one hand, that can be something literal like a dark energy, it can be any thought, belief, or emotion. Most people might associate that with what they might evaluate as a negative emotion like anger. But falling in love could also qualify as a superimposition because it can take you over. Any ideology or identity that turns fanatical can qualify.

While Superimposition Patterns manifest in a variety of ways, we particularly wanted to include the following two sessions. They are deeply compelling, and the implications of each of them are very far-reaching in very different ways. Most other Superimposition Pattern stories and the implication of their release, while highly significant to our clients who experienced them, are much less dramatic and earth shattering in general.

Case One: Demons Get Inside

Jean is a highly functioning, professional woman in her mid-forties who came for treatment with several presenting physical symptoms and a particularly disturbing and unusual experience. For a month, she had had increasing sleep disturbances, a sense of tightness in her chest, and constriction in her throat. She couldn't find a way to quiet herself internally, which had always been relatively easy for her. Jean had noted these symptoms, and while many were quite unusual for her, she could find a way to explain all of them separately and circumstantially. For example, her recent visit to her childhood home could spark trouble sleeping and a bit of anxiety to create tightness in her chest, and seasonal allergies and asthma could absolutely cause tightness in her chest and constriction in her throat. None of the symptoms, in and of themselves, were sufficient for Jean to initiate making an appointment for therapy.

Then one day, while on a lunch break from work, Jean took a walk down the street and saw a pubescent twelve-year-old girl walking by. As Jean saw the girl, she heard a voice in her head say, "Look at those titties!" The voice had a licentious tone and feel. This was so upsetting and unfamiliar to Jean that she immediately called for a session. When she came in, she had no sense that the voice and the symptoms of the previous month were related. The predatory experience was so repulsive and disturbing that she was shaken to her core. Jean was heterosexual and had never before had any attraction to females, never mind young girls. While she had been a victim of sexual violence, she had never experienced herself as a predator. In fact, harmony was very important to her.

As the session progressed, Jean's deepest wisdom through the muscle testing indicated that all of the physical symptoms and the voice itself were all manifestations of one organizing difficulty that we call a *Superimposition*. It further indicated that while the Superimposition originated about a month prior, it had nothing to do with her trip to her family of origin, the event that Jean had most associated with the onset of the physical symptoms. Instead, we discovered that the root cause occurred just prior to her trip.

Since muscle testing had indicated that the pattern involved was a Superimposition, Jean used the statement, "Something much bigger than me has taken me over." She focused on the most disturbing body sensation, an agitation so large that it felt as if she couldn't live in her own skin. As she brought all of her consciousness to this sensation, she saw herself a month ago having sexual intercourse with her lover, a policeman who had been involved with the case of a pedophile, though the officer had not spoken to her about it at the time. Focusing on the sensation, she realized that this was the moment the Superimposition entered her, and it could account for all the symptoms.

Muscle testing called for Jean to channel gold Light. Opening to this Light, Jean reported that she felt bathed in this Light and felt a sense of rebalancing. She then brought all of her attention to each of her chakras, starting at the root and holding each in their typical color within the gold Light. She reported that that night she slept normally with all the other symptoms gone by the following morning. Jean has been symptom free since and all the lascivious desire for girls just disappeared.

Jean speculated that her lover was carrying this energy because of his ongoing proximity to pedophiles and when they were being intimate, it gained access to her. This session is compelling in that it opens us to the question of whether some pedophilic perpetrators are sitting with a Superimposition Pattern, an energy that takes them over, and they lack the resilience to recognize and contain it and not take destructive action in the world.

Sometimes, a Superimposition can appear in nightmares.

One session felt particularly important, given that it involved confronting years of unrelenting nightmares which had begun to have serious effects on my mental health. In these dreams, I would witness a myriad of gruesome events happening to me and my loved ones. During the session, I was guided to a demon-like Superimposition clinging to my soul and spirit. Through a series of movements, I finally broke its hold, and, with it, an unforgettable, lasting sense of relief and wholeness washed over me. Since this session years ago, I have had only a few of these nightmares, and their effects on me have been greatly diminished.

—Elan Green

Case Two: Shattered

Joy had been hospitalized several times for threatening suicide and not being able to care for herself. At times, she had a full range of what are typically described as delusions, hallucinations, and all of the symptoms of what is currently called dissociative identity disorder (DID). Specifically, there were gaps of times that she could not account for; she had different personalities with different names, and she believed that bugs were crawling on her body, even though she knew that that seemed impossible. She had been hospitalized many times for these problems and had been on various psychotropic medications, but nothing had helped. She reported a history that is typical in such cases and that could account for her symptoms. A hellacious history, she reported verbal, physical, and sexual abuse in childhood, and, perhaps worst of all, she witnessed her sister's murder.

Muscle testing revealed that the most important thing to work on was her DID. It went on to reveal something quite extraordinary—that the root of the DID was none of the traumatic experiences she had shared about her life. Rather, the root cause of Joy's dissociative identity disorder was a Superimposition Pattern. Joy spontaneously blurted out that this made total sense. She reported that thirty years prior to the session, when she was eight years old, she was at a Southern Baptist Fundamentalist Church service. During the "fire and brimstone" sermon, a dark energy took her over. She was already in therapy at that point. When she next went to her psychiatrist and told him about this, she reported that her psychiatrist said that she needed medication and put her on Thorazine. She vowed in that moment that she would never tell anybody about her experience again.

Muscle testing next revealed that the memory was, in fact, where the current symptoms associated with the DID diagnosis had begun. Muscle testing further revealed that Joy knew what she had to do to release the Superimposition. At that point, Joy gave Andy a look that implied that the suggestion that she knew what to do was crazy. Still, just a moment later, her eyes brightened, and she stood up. "I need to do a Native American dance," she said, adding, "even though I'm only one-sixteenth Native American, and I have no idea how to do it."

After she found the sensation associated with the Superimposition and let the eight-year-old tell her story of what it was like being taken over, she started to do a very intricate dance. About a minute into it, she looked up as if to say, "What am I doing?" and then continued the dance. A short while later, it was as though both she and Andy could almost feel the room shake and brighten, and she looked up and said, "It's done."

While Andy continued to see Joy for a few years after this session, and even though she still suffered greatly, there was a very noticeable decrease in her symptoms immediately after that session, and it seemed that her clinical course had been altered. She began to develop a better observing ego, sense of self, witness function, and access to her Higher Self as described in many healing traditions. Andy happened to run into Joy twenty-five years later, and she was happy to report she had never been hospitalized since their work together.

While we certainly are not implying that all dissociative identity disorders with psychotic features are caused by dark Superimpositions, it certainly seems to have had a profound effect in this case, and it does intuitively make some sense. Because, in our clinical experience, when dark Superimpositions tend to take over a person, people can feel like they have lost their observing ego and their capacity to hold themselves together. It's as if all of the different multiple beings who inhabit the community of our Soul can take over with no functioning executive running the show.

Extraterrestrials

Extraterrestrials (from the Latin *extra*—beyond or not of, and *terrestris* —of or belonging to Earth) are defined as life that does not originate from Earth. They are often referred to as aliens. In the context of this system, the Extraterrestrial Pattern refers to energies that can create up to four different experiences in a person. In the first three of these forms, the person usually identifies as being human, while in the fourth, the person identifies as an extraterrestrial in a story. More specifically, the first three forms include: (1) implants—energetic structures implanted into the person for the purposes of experimentation/control; (2) abduction—a sense of being taken against one's will with all the accompanying senses of violation and impotency; and (3) walk-ins—a sense that some other life force has entered the person's body, is using it, and may have pushed the person into the background or off to the side. In the fourth instance, the person identifies with the extraterrestrial life form rather than the human form, and various themes can arise. These themes include and are not limited to: (1) a loss of sense of home with a potential to feel an obligation to leave home in order to accomplish a mission; (2) journeys going awry; (3) an overemphasis on the mind at the expense of the heart; or (4) a sense of being a stranger in a strange land.

To reiterate once again, a key in these stories is theme. In one session, muscle testing revealed an experience of an Extraterrestrial Implant that further diagnosis revealed to represent an experience with a cult. That information was very useful in the healing. Any story in which a person is taken against their will can map, present, or be perceived as an abduction. Anytime it feels like another being has become so powerful in your life that it is like you are speaking their thoughts, it can be mapped or represented as a walk-in. And anytime you feel alienated in a way that makes you experience life as truly an outsider, it can map/present as you being a traumatized extraterrestrial.

A Case: I Don't Want to Hear; Ringing in the Ear

John had been bothered by tinnitus and hearing loss in one ear for many years. Doctors found no obvious cause, and John knew of no obvious precipitant. Muscle testing again revealed that the tinnitus was related to an Extraterrestrial Implant Pattern. Like so many others, John was skeptical. Nonetheless, when he brought his attention to the implant, he could feel a density in his head near his ear. Focusing on the energy, he realized that there was something he very much was afraid he would hear and did not want to. He had subliminally put out a prayer to the Universe to protect him from hearing it. John then saw a strange creature putting something rod-like in his ear. He realized he had to ask the creature to come back and remove the rod. He did this, and the creature honored his request, and John felt the rod melting. John reported that that night, his wife whispered something in his ear, and he actually could hear a little in that ear.

This session reveals something that we've witnessed on several occasions. When a client doesn't want to hear something (especially about themselves), it can literally affect their hearing. The same has come up in sessions concerning difficulties with vision. Often, these involve clients who literally didn't want to see something visually or perceive something emotionally.

I woke from a nightmare in the middle of the night, startled and agitated. My husband turned to me and asked what was wrong. "I know it's crazy," I said, "but I had a dream that I was abducted by aliens, and they were doing things to my reproductive tract." My husband immediately turned on the light and said seriously, "I just had the exact same dream." We frantically discussed the scene in the dream—we were both lying down on tables next to each other, and aliens were inserting threadlike instruments into our bodies. Our dreams were identical. As scientists (my husband is a microbiologist, and I was a biochemical researcher for a pharmaceutical company at the time), we had no logical, scientific explanation for our experience. Believe me when I tell you that we were both very aware of how f***ing weird it was! We're scientists! We resolved that we'd never tell anyone about it; it was just too f***ing crazy.

Then, we started to get weird symptoms that our medical doctors couldn't explain, and we had more of the abduction nightmares. My husband got headaches, chronic fatigue no matter how much sleep he got, and blood in his semen—that was scary. The doctors told him that nothing was wrong; he was totally healthy. And he wasn't an athlete and didn't work out in any way that could cause damage in that area. As for me, I stopped menstruating and developed rashes, headaches, anxiety, depression, exhaustion, extreme pain in my groin, and an overall feeling of not feeling like myself. My medical doctors had no logical medical explanation for my symptoms either. Every time I went to my gynecologist, she asked if I'd been raped or molested because anytime she touched me, I freaked out. I swore on my life multiple times that I'd never been abused, and I have not been. Then, I felt like something was inside of me. Multiple pregnancy tests came back negative. But it gets even weirder. One day, I had an experience in a bathroom stall at work that I can only describe as a miscarriage. There was so much blood, and the pain was indescribable.

As our symptoms worsened, my husband and I were running out of medical specialists to go to, and we were no closer to a diagnosis for either one of us. We were both asking who in the world we could go to for help. We intuitively felt that our symptoms were connected to our shared abduction nightmares. And again, we were fully aware of how f***ing crazy that sounds! I finally confided in my best friend about what was going on. She connected me with Andy and Life Centered Therapy.

In two sessions with Andy, our physical symptoms disappeared— poof and gone. Andy gave us the space to tell our story and to really go back to the nightmares and focus there. The key to healing for us was (1) acknowledgment of the trauma, and (2) creating boundaries by gaining the empowerment to say, "No! You're no longer going to do things to me without my consent." Neither my husband nor I have had an abduction nightmare again, and our physical symptoms have not returned.

—Erica Barnes

Another woman rediscovered the magic of joy in her life and was able to leave an unfulfilling job and move to a more fulfilling career path with confidence after resolving her abduction experience. This experience revealed itself to her in a story not about extraterrestrials, but about a man abducting a fairy in the forest—and with her playing the role of the fairy. Remember that any story in which a person is taken against their will can map, present, or be *perceived* as an abduction.

There was a heaviness weighing on me, an underlying fear that even though things were feeling good, at any moment, the rug could be ripped out from underneath me, and I'd be left with nothing.

In an LCT session, the journey of the day brought me to another lifetime, in which I was a woodland nymph. Bouncing from rock to rock along the banks of a river, I left a trail of what I can only describe as magical pixie dust behind me. Joy, magic, and connection with the land around me oozed from every pore of my little nymph body. There was a deep interconnection with the water, the rocks, the sunshine, the squirrels and chipmunks, and every single plant around me. I was light and free, moving through the world with joy and ease until I felt the presence of another being, a human in the forest. Before I could get away, I was snatched up in a net and tied up in a cloth sack. In that moment, fear and panic took over, and the connection with the land was severed like a cut from a knife. Thrashing around inside of the bag and trying to get out only led to exhaustion. The magic inside of me was depleted, getting thrown from my body with every shake.

After what seemed like eternity, the bag opened, and I was tossed inside of a wooden cell where there were other magical creatures— fairies, nymphs, and elves. I wasn't sure where exactly this place was, but the one thing that was certain was that we were there for the entertainment of these humans who had captured us all. But, because all of our magic was pulled from us, being disconnected from the land and all that animates us, there was no way we could put on a show full of magic like we were expected to. Because of that, the humans used torture as a method to make us conform to what they wanted.

I was beaten down physically, emotionally, energetically, again and again and again, for what seemed like an eternity—until the realization came one day that I could bring my mind and my Soul to the woods. I could connect with that place inside of me as if I were there in real life. It was not dissociation; it was a real connection. It started as a faint whisper, but the more I focused, the more that connection grew. Before long, I could feel that joy and magic as if it was right in front of me, even though my physical body was still being tortured and beaten down.

Everything from there on was a blur. Very quickly, I found within me the courage to formulate a plan for escape, and before I could process what had happened, I found myself back on the river where I once lived, frolicking once again on the rocks along the water, singing with the birds and the plants. But it was even more beautiful than I remembered. I could feel the sun singing, singing deep into my bones. The plants were infusing me with a life and a love in a way that is indescribable.

Processing that experience in my waking life after the session shifted my fundamental view of the world. The heaviness I felt in my chest had lifted. The flowers looked brighter. My body was lighter. LCT helped me to remember that we hold the magic within us, always.

—Caroline

Conclusion

We have just shared with you an introduction to the nonmaterial patterns. While we have not illustrated all of the variations of nonmaterial realm patterns, these are a good representative sample. Our hope was to not only familiarize you with the patterns, but also to illustrate their usefulness in healing. For those who have had these types of experiences and understand them in this way, we hope you have found a sense of acceptance and deeper understanding. For those who have had these experiences yet have not known how to understand them, we hope the information provides a sense of relief and comfort in the knowledge gained. For those who are wary and deeply skeptical, we hope you feel held in your skepticism while being invited into opening to possibilities that can create deeper understanding of yours and others' experiences without feeling a sense of being coerced. For those who have never thought about it, we hope you feel a sense of excitement about exploring these concepts further so that you know your own truth about how you feel about them and what place they might hold in your personal meaning-making.

We, as the authors, each have our personal ideas on the literalness of these phenomena, and from a professional perspective, our personal ideas are irrelevant. In a similar fashion, we believe that our clients' beliefs are not for us to evaluate and only matter to us insofar as they affect their capacity to heal. What is significant is how useful the application of the themes is to our clients. As you can see, we have a great deal of experience that teaches us that working with these themes unquestionably helps to alleviate people's suffering. The themes are an important part of our healing tool bag. Our hope is that this introduction is useful to you in your healing journey.

CHAPTER 10

When We Protect Ourselves and That Becomes the Problem

In this chapter, we're going to spell out in much greater detail problems that are not the reenactment of a trauma but the reenactment of the way that we choose to protect ourselves from ever having to experience a trauma again. Recall, in Chapter 5, we made a distinction between what caused Sylvia and Nate's depressions. Sylvia was reenacting a trauma while Nate was reenacting how he responded to the trauma.

To give another simple example of reliving the trauma versus reliving the protection we choose in the wake of the trauma, suppose that we are agoraphobic, meaning that we can't leave our house. If we are reliving a trauma, we may be stuck in a story in which we were put in a prison, gave up all hope of escape, and lived a very constricted, barren life. Alternatively, if we are reliving a protector story that we chose without awareness, we may have a story in which we raced out into the street in pursuit of a ball when we were a small child and nearly got run over by a bus. In our terror, we raced back into our house as a way of protecting ourselves from our fear of death. Clearly, that was a good choice at the time. The problem is that we live the limitation of the choice in circumstances that are similar but do not call for that choice.

In this example, anytime we feel the call of chasing our dreams, we will feel threatened, and we may literally or figuratively end up housebound for no apparent reason, particularly if we have repressed the early-in-life incident. Even, however, if we do remember the original incident, until we realize that our symptom is, in fact, a protector that we chose to have come in without realizing we were making a choice, we will be stuck automatically making the same choice, even when we know it profoundly limits us and can make us miserable.

Pragmatically, how we make sense of our lives is vitally important. And understanding how something that has plagued us as a problem is actually something that we brought in to protect ourselves at a different time can give us a whole new perspective of the problem. This means that, in fact, upon reflection, we can be appreciative and ultimately even grateful.

Healing Problems That Are Protectors

The key to healing this pattern is, first, to realize that the current symptom is a reliving of a choice that we made that was the best choice we could have made at the time. The problem is that because we were traumatized, we lose perspective and automatically make the choice without awareness. Because of this, the choice has become generalized to our lives and limits us. It's what creates the problem that makes us seek help.

When we are working with this pattern, it brings our awareness to the limiting choice way back when. From a place of fear, we did not have the discernment to not generalize it to every similar circumstance in our lives, and that is the limitation. We can decide if we now want to make a different choice to release the limitation of the choice that served originally but no longer does.

Invariably, we do. In this case, we can thank the protector and tell it we no longer need it. How do we release it? We can literally just bring all of our attention to the body sensation associated with the protector and use our consciousness to move it from inside ourselves to outside ourselves. We can imagine it; we can use our hands; or we can just do it in the blink of an eye. Since we chose to ask it to come in, we can choose to ask it to go out.

Once we have externalized the energy of the young, traumatized person and the protector, we choose to become a channel of Source energy, bringing Source Light through us to the dense energy until it is totally infused with the Light. This is a practice that can heal the original trauma. We can discover if this has made any difference in our relationship to the original traumatic scene and what lessons we can learn about how "the problem" has helped us.

We ought to feel more spacious inside. The truer self can be found in that spaciousness where it had been hiding or hidden for all this time, waiting for us to rediscover and reclaim it. This is actually easy to do. All we have to do is find the true self, put our hands lovingly on our body where we sense it has been hiding/hidden, and invite it to come out and touch our hand and expand forward and back, left and right, and up and down until it fills us to overflowing. Then, we get to experience all of who we were before we made the choice, and incorporate all of the experiences that we've had since then.

A Deeper Understanding of What Happens: Introjection

Now that we have talked about the basic problem and the way we can heal it, let's turn to a fuller understanding. When we have a traumatic experience where we make an automatic choice to protect ourselves, the first thing that happens, to use a term in psychology, is to *introject*, or to take in the entire traumatic experience. *Introjection* is a process in which an individual unconsciously incorporates aspects of external reality, in this case, the traumatic event, into the self, particularly when there are powerful mixed feelings (for example, when you love the person, and you hate and are overwhelmed by the way they are treating you in a particular situation).

Holding inside of you the entire experience of the traumatic event can serve in several ways: (1) to gain control of the situation by bringing it inside you; (2) to be able to heal the trauma that arises from the experience without having to do it in the external world, particularly with the person who traumatized you; and/or (3) to give you options around protecting yourself by allowing you to choose the best mechanism to keep you safe, including minimizing the likelihood that the traumatic event will ever happen again.

The first thing that happens when we take in the scene is that we literally start acting out the interaction inside of ourselves, meaning we act out a reaction to the introjected aggressor in order to protect ourselves. For example, suppose your father calls you stupid when you're trying to help him out, and you can't handle his reaction. You might begin to call yourself stupid when you're trying to accomplish something. It will sound like your voice to you, but in reality, it's your father's voice that you have taken in. In reaction, you will have one of three responses: fight, flight, or freeze. If you fight, you might internally tell them to go f*** themselves or be passive-aggressive and say to yourself, *You can't control me, I will do nothing.* If you take flight, you might keep that voice at bay by passively cowering and being paralyzed with anxiety, or placate that voice by being ingratiating. If you freeze, you don't feel. Think of Nate saying, "I don't care."

Everything we experience internally, we unconsciously project onto our outer world and create situations that look similar. This is the reason that we live the limitation of that earlier choice we made to protect ourselves.

This was all very complicated. We are now going to give you a way to map out what is actually happening. This will make it easier to understand and track the experience.

An Overview of Protecting Identities

These protection stories play out on four different levels. The first level is the context in which the protection occurs. This is called *Structure*. The second level is *Role*. The third is *Behavior*. The fourth is *Shadow*. Let us explain.

Structure

Structure concerns the context in which the protection occurs. It can be in a two-person relationship where one of the people is you; we call this *dyadic*. It can occur in any larger system of which you are a part. The primary system is the family, and there are obviously numerous other systems in which we are all involved. We call this *systemic*. It can also occur when we take in another relationship which we witness, even though we are not directly involved in it. By far, the most common of these is our parents' relationship. We call this *relational*.

Role: Parallel/Reversed

Role concerns whether, in a future situation, we replay the role that we played in the original situation, or we replay the role of someone(s) who was/were in relationship with us. If we replay our own role, we call this *parallel*. If we replay the role of someone(s) who is/are in relationship with us, we call this *reversed*.

Behavior: Parallel/Reversed

We can either behave in the same way we or the person/people we were involved with behaved. We call this parallel. Or we can behave in exactly the opposite way we or the people we were involved with behaved. We call this reversed.

Shadow

This last level concerns our inability to accept some aspect of ourselves, so we are judgmental of it. Finding it unacceptable in ourselves, we seek out versions of it in other people and then, instead of dealing with our own lack of self-acceptance, we project the quality onto them and then judge it and attack it in them. We call this Shadow. A particularly virulent example of this is when we do this with our children.

Blocked Identity Dyadic Examples

In this explanation, we break down three scenarios: one in which the person's protection aligns with the victim, the second in which the protection aligns with the perpetrator, and the third in which the protection aligns internally with the victim and the perpetrator.

Aligning with the Victim

Nate's case is an example of a dyadic structure (he and his father) with a parallel role (Nate in adulthood is in the same role as Nate as a young boy), and parallel behavior (Nate says, "I don't care," in both instances).

If you recall, in Nate's story, we discovered that having his father not accept his gift, push him away, walk off, and drive away was too painful for Nate to bear. Instead of experiencing the excruciating pain of feeling rejected and abandoned in this way, Nate unconsciously chose to protect his truer creative, exuberant, buoyant self by hiding it, and keeping it hidden, behind a numbing protector whose identity is "I don't care." Nate aligned with the victim as a way of protecting himself.

Apparently, this was the best choice Nate could have made at the time. The problem is that because he made such a choice during a time of trauma, he unwittingly generalized it to any situation that bore a resemblance to that day, almost like his identity was frozen in that originating moment. In Nate's case, this meant that whenever he felt the possibility of being abandoned and not being received, he unconsciously hid and continued to hide behind an obscuring protective limiting identity, the identity that we might call "I don't care."

It's only when we consciously realize that what we believe to be a problem is, in fact, a choice we made to call in a protector to protect ourselves from a worse problem, that we can thank the protector, acknowledge their service, wake the chooser up, so to speak, and consciously make a different choice to let the protector go.

We do this by bringing the energy of the traumatized one (the young

Nate) and the protector (the choice to not feel, who we called "I don't care") outside ourselves. Then, heal the traumatized one and the protector by infusing them with Source Light. Finally, allow the untraumatized one (Nate before he made the limiting choice) to come forward.

Aligning with the Perpetrator

We are still with Nate and his father (dyadic), but this time we are going to look at reversed roles (if Nate had taken on his father's role), with parallel behavior (Nate taking on his father's behavior).

In this scenario, Nate could have protected himself in the story by aligning with his father's experience—to identify with the person who was aggressive toward him. Nate protects himself by covering over his exuberant, creative, buoyant, truer self with an abandoning, withdrawing energy—the energy he experienced coming from his father to him. (Remember that Nate has already taken the whole experience inside himself; so, he has access to acting like his father.)

Needing the approval and love of his father, Nate would be willing to take on the bad behavior to protect his truer self by unconsciously choosing to become exactly like his father. This choice would also protect Nate just like "I don't care" protected Nate, mainly because identifying with and acting like his father would equally hide the truer and more innocent self. Secondarily, it might protect Nate because it allows him to continue to stay close to his father by being like him. This explains the possibility of Nate, when he becomes a parent, treating his child the way he was treated and provides one possible explanation of why some people who were abused as children end up abusing in the same way they were abused.

If Nate had chosen to protect himself in this way, his symptom may have presented differently from the depression that emerged when his protector aligned with himself as the victim. In the case of Nate's protector aligning with his father, Nate may have come in for therapy because he was having trouble in his intimate relationship. Every time his partner reached out lovingly with an actual gift, a gift of service, or warmth, Nate may have not been able to receive it. And if Nate had repressed the whole original situation, he would have no idea why this was so. Even if he hadn't fully repressed the original scene, he still would not know how to make a different choice.

In our diagnostic, we might discover that his intention is a Blocked Identity where the context is dyadic, the role is reversed, and the behavior is parallel. At this point, we can share with Nate that his behavior is a protection, and it's not even *his* protection—it's taking on his father's role as protection.

In this scenario, Nate will feel the sensations associated with abandoning and withdrawing. When he discovers the sensations and becomes them, he will discover the original story. He will then be able to cast out the protector and the energy from the original trauma and heal his trauma with Source Light as described above. Then, he will be free of the original trauma and able to make more conscious choices about how to proceed when faced with similar situations in his life.

Aligning Internally with Perpetrator *and* Victim

In life, Nate might exactly replicate in his internal world what he experienced with his father in the outer world. To give but one possibility, Nate could start abandoning the creative exuberant gift-giver and walk away from his own creations and/or find them unacceptable in his own eyes, and then shut down and get depressed, internally playing out both sides as an exact replica of what happened externally.

This introjecting still protects Nate by keeping the problem internalized so that he controls it, *and* it ensures that Nate will never lose connection with his parent. In this way, it allows for the possibility to transform the whole dynamic if Nate comes to realize what has happened. Nate can then internally resolve it without having to depend on anyone else or anyone else's maturing. It is remarkable what we will unconsciously do to maintain our relationship with the parent and our capacity to potentially heal that relationship even at great expense.

Blocked Identities: Systemic

Sometimes the context where we experience the trauma is not between us and one other person; the trauma occurs in the context of a system. The system may be our family, our professional work group, or any system that we define. In this case, the protector who we unconsciously choose can be: (1) the role we play in the system in order to keep it balanced and secure; (2) the role any, some, or all the other people play in relationship to us; or (3) all roles.

Case One: Dulling Her Shine

A woman came in for a session because she was presenting with the following physical symptoms: fatigue, foggy memory, a pounding headache, dizziness, sleepiness, hair loss, and acid reflux.

Muscle testing indicated that her highest priority intention was every thing she said, and it further revealed that all of her symptoms were a Blocked Identity. I was therefore able to tell Pamela that what she called her fatigue, foggy memory, pounding headache, dizziness, sleepiness, hair loss, and acid reflux was, in fact, *a choice* that she had made at an earlier time. While this was the best choice she could have made at the time, it was now limiting her tremendously. Pamela understood what I was saying but could not consciously relate it to any event in her life.

Muscle testing revealed that she made this choice at age thirty-nine. Pamela immediately exclaimed, "Oh, I know what this is...a memory just came to me that I haven't thought about in years. At every job I had in my thirties, I was shining, performing very well, getting lots of positive feedback and attention from upper management, but every immediate boss I had resented it."

"It seemed as if they were insecure, and it felt like they wanted me to be quiet and not so outspoken. And I know what this mask/protection is ... There was this moment when I said, 'I want to lay low, not shine...it's more agony than it's worth.'"

Muscle testing confirmed that this was in fact the obscuring identity. At this point in the session, Pamela began to have a strange sensation in her throat and began to burp. She also felt a throbbing in the palm of her hand, headache, fogginess in head, and pounding in her stomach. Bringing all her attention and awareness to the sensations, she said, "I was at the last job I had in my thirties as part of a small startup, and a new higher-up, right off the bat, came into the company and started letting people go. I was one of them even though I was top performer and getting excellent reviews. I was shocked, considering how well I was doing in every aspect of the job." Pamela further commented, "As I was leaving, I was so enraged that I told the VP that this new executive was an asshole; he treated me terribly, and I didn't deserve this decision. I didn't care about his reference, and I stormed out of the company."

Continuing her story, Pamela explained, "I was unemployed for about twelve months and suffered quite a bit during that time. After that, it felt like I had learned not to shine too brightly...and in my next jobs for the next twenty years or so, while I was a strong performer and content with my work life, I was no longer the superstar I used to be. Intuitively it feels that I was afraid on some deeper level that I could have that same situation happen again if I performed at too high a level and was as outspoken as I had been. It feels like there is a block around speaking my truth, some kind of protection in my throat. It also feels relevant that I had been struggling for years to get a promotion at my new job until I just recently finally got promoted."

Muscle testing revealed that we had to dialogue with this identity about the history of its relationship with Pamela, and how it served/limited her. She asked the identity how it served her, protected her, and limited her. The following came to her awareness:

"It protected me . . . it made me forget that the event had ever happened because I had taken it too personally at the time. It also limited me in that it let diseases drive me . . . I've been consumed with several diseases over the past two decades that have been keeping me away from work, always been on my mind, and sucking my energy and happiness. I've never been able to understand where all these diseases came from."

I invited Pamela to use her imagination to place the image of that scene across the room and to make a different choice about her physical symptoms and decision to lay low and not shine. I invited her to externalize the choice and the traumatized one.

I asked her to tell me what she saw outside herself. "A dark swirling black energy." Pamela infused it with Light. "I need to send it back to the Divine," she said. She proceeded to do so with her imagination and reported that she now felt a sense of lightness. I invited Pamela to go into the newfound lightness and find her true self that had been obscured and was hiding under what had been the dark swirling black energy.

As she did this, she said she saw a beautiful glowing orange/yellow light that felt like her true self who is kind, nonjudgmental, happy to serve others, full of ideas, loves to share these ideas freely, and enjoys working and creating. Pamela let this expand throughout her body. She announced that she felt like a new person and all the throbbing in palm, pounding in stomach, fogginess in head, dizziness, and low energy were gone. She had a sense of aliveness and lightness that felt incredible.

We found that all these symptoms had an energetic component to them that were manifesting themselves physically. By doing work on the energetic root cause, in the days following the session she was able to find more relief than she had found before. Interestingly, she also mentioned that her main concern about her hair loss was that it was going to lead her to be neglected for promotions and advancement in her company due to ageism, which aligns with the notion that the protection was to prevent career advancement due to past trauma.

Furthermore, while she had been battling these physical symptoms in varying levels of intensity for the past twenty years, they increased dramatically in severity two weeks before the session. Pamela made the connection that she was finally promoted two weeks earlier after years of consciously trying to achieve this, and felt a literal shock run through her body when she got the news. She was stunned at that moment, and it was a strange sensation she had never had before, although she was of course simultaneously overjoyed to have finally been promoted.

In the days following the promotion, all her symptoms got noticeably worse. She had already been working with Tibetan medicine and Western medicine to manage her symptoms, and they didn't appear to be able to help her symptoms in the past weeks as well as they had in the long run.

Since this protection of "wanting to lay low, not shine" was still active when she was recently promoted, it's as if the second she got promoted, it was the ultimate threat to this protection. She would be in a higher position in her company, in the limelight, which may have resulted in the same trauma happening again to her. This may explain why seemingly out of the blue, her hair loss got worse, her acid reflux intensified, and she began getting headaches, having more fatigue, and increasing memory problems. This all happened on one level, in order to protect her even more intensely from a perceived threat.

Pamela's experience in the days after the session:

It has now been five days since my session. The rate of my hair loss has noticeably decreased; I no longer wake up with hair all over my pillow. This to me is a miracle. My headaches that came out of the blue a few weeks ago and had been consistent until the session, have not returned. The dizziness is also completely gone, and I feel a significant boost in energy. I have spent years working on treating the physical symptoms with both Western and Eastern medicine and never would have thought they were (in part) a psychospiritual protection . . . I am truly amazed and hopeful that this healing will last.

I went to a wedding this weekend and met lots of new people. I had amazing conversations that I initiated, and I felt noticeably more confident in myself with no hesitation in my speech. In the past, I always hesitated to talk to people . . . but at this wedding, I wasn't alone for a single moment, and it was with people I had never met before. Not feeling self-conscious was a totally new experience for me. My heart feels open and full. I can't remember the last time I have ever felt this way.

Pamela's experience two weeks after the session:

I have been on 50 mcg of thyroid meds for a number of years. This has always kept my thyroid hormone levels in the right range. A month and a half ago, I had my TSH level tested, which is one of the main hormonal indicators of hypothyroidism. It was 7.1, indicating that my medication dosage was no longer sufficient. I did not want to increase the dosage of the meds, so I waited. I just did a blood test recently and received my TSH level, and it is now on the low end of normal. It is the lowest it has ever been since I started taking meds, and I am still remaining symptom free and feel transformed on the levels of mind, body, and spirit.

Case Two: Sickness as Savior

Fred came in for treatment because of ongoing physical sickness that seemed to have no obvious medical cause. Fred noticed that this had happened intermittently before but had become a real problem when he moved to Boston from Southern California to take a new job. His gut reaction was that it was precipitated by the move and the change of climate.

Muscle testing revealed that his sicknesses equaled a protection where the structure was systemic, and the role and behavior were parallel (the same he played out earlier). When Fred dropped into the sensation associated with sickness and became it, he started to replay a very vivid scene. In the scene, his family was having a terrible fight. It literally made him feel sick, and he started to have severe nausea and chills. Fred's experience was that, as soon as he got sick, the fighting stopped, and he got lots of attention and loving care. He laughingly said that his sickness had saved the day. He then saw further scenes with his family where the same pattern occurred. No one recognized the relationship between the family fights and Fred getting sick.

When Fred continued to feel the sickness as a sensation in the body and moved into the present, he realized that the same thing was happening at work. In his old job, there was an easy-going, harmonious atmosphere. In his new job, there were many disagreements among coworkers and tensions ran high. Fred hated the tension and had the sense that when he got sick, it lessened the amount of chaos and conflict he experienced at work. Secondarily, it got him attention, commiseration, and support.

When Fred found his truer self and embodied it, he felt a sense of vitality that he said had been missing in his life. Several weeks later, Fred was surprised but happy to report that he had felt fine for the last several weeks and that he looked forward to that continuing.

The above story points out one more thing that is very important as we do our healing work in our own systems. It is so often the case that someone is called the problem (Fred getting sick) as opposed to the realization that there is an underlying problem that is determined by the whole system (family fighting all the time). In the field of psychology, this person (Fred) is typically called "the identified patient." Invariably, not only is the role they play in the system not acknowledged, but people who play this role are typically labeled "sick" or "bad." Perhaps a truer statement of the situation is that they're the most sensitive people in the system and act like "canaries in the coal mine," harbingers of unrealized danger who are sacrificed as a way to keep the larger system safe.

When we stop seeing someone as the problem, in this case Fred who is always getting sick, and realize that there *is* a problem, that the family is fighting a lot in potentially destructive ways, which Fred's sensitivity may have a role in, whole new possibilities become available to address the true cause of the difficulties. It's not that anyone is just reacting; everyone is co-creating the difficulties that arise. Everybody's perception of their role in the system and the dynamic in the system can be revealed and acknowledged. And once the underlying difficulties are revealed, everyone can become a member of a team, working together to find the best resolutions.

In this way, each member of the system becomes a participant in the healing process. And when this happens, remarkably, people no longer need to stay stuck in rigid roles. They can begin to embody their true selves in an environment that is not only safer, but that actively supports this.

Blocked Identity; Relational

The protector in the relational structure does not arise out of something that was overtly directed at you, but something you witnessed, typically your parents' relationship. Let's suppose when you were very young, you witnessed your parents fighting, and you were afraid that they would get divorced and that you would lose one or both of them. One way to protect yourself from this fear of abandonment would be to take their relationship inside yourself, to literally introject their relationship so that no matter what happens, you will always have them with you. Then, even if you literally lose your parents or figuratively lose them because of the pain you experience in witnessing their relationship, on a whole other level, you get to control the fact that they will never internally leave you.

The problem, however, is that in this circumstance, the template you have for relationship is engraved in you, not just a way of relating that is familiar to you. This engraving can affect you at any time. As you enter a relationship yourself, you may unknowingly use this template in your own relationship as a way to try to heal the trauma you felt witnessing your parents' relationship. In your internal experience, you need to have their relationship survive and thrive.

What can be challenging about this is that sometimes we may have a relationship that is going very well and then, when we get married, trouble arises. The reason this happens is that the trauma is associated specifically with marriage and doesn't rear its ugly head, so to speak, until you put yourself in the same place as your parents by getting married.

As with any pattern of this type, healing begins when you realize that you have internalized this pattern as a way of protecting yourself and trying to heal your trauma from your parents' relationship. In this case, what you are externalizing is the traumatized younger you and the parents' dysfunctional relationship. So, when you channel Light into this, you heal the younger you, and you realize that taking in the parents' relationship actually protected you, which can change your perception of the relationship itself.

Then, you'll be able to go into the spaciousness that is now in the body and find the truer you who knows intuitively what a good relationship can be like. You can invite that energy to expand in all directions until it fills you to overflowing. Invariably, then you can imagine what you want in a relationship, and your relationship to yourself can improve as well as your relationship with others.

Today, I feel the tension in my right hip, and the pull from my right side to the left along my pelvis, horizontal to my body. The right side pulls tightly from my neck all the way down to my knee. It feels tightly wound, tense, inflamed, angry, and about to explode. I hear myself describing my father in my childhood. The left side of my body seems calm and relaxed in comparison, ignoring the pulling from the right, as if it has its back turned, not experiencing or witnessing the pain and ignoring the obvious torquing of the other side. My mother is represented by the left side. It's as if I have taken them in physically, not my parents themselves, but the tension and the structure of their relationship, and recreated it in my body. Perhaps my body wanted me to remember something it knew I had forgotten. Perhaps it wanted me to heal from the past. Maybe this was the only way I knew to stay safe, or I may have thought it was my job to repair them. I have always been in the middle in a way, as the middle child, and now, as an adult, I feel stuck in the middle of this tension in my body.

I visualize placing this heavy energy from my pelvis outside my body. I use "boundary tapping" [see Chapter 14] to brush it up and out, and I feel a shift after a few minutes, a lightness in my lower torso, a feeling of slightly more room and less pain. I go back inside and visualize the moment that I chose to take in that layer of protection, a little girl who felt stuck in the middle, trapped in family dynamics. I then place my hands out in front of me, palms up, envisioning my younger self inside that layer of energy that I have removed, like a child in a gray ball resting on top of my outstretched hands. I send her love, forgiveness, and gratitude. My eyes have been closed for most of the session, and I continue that way, envisioning myself in my childhood bedroom wrapped in positive energy.

As instructed, I go back inside one more time, but this time I find the girl I was before I took in that protection. I see myself outside on a blanket as a two-year-old, unaware of others and my limitations, standing up to a little boy teasing me. I put my hand on my abdomen and imagine taking her inside myself, filling up the space left there by the removal of the old, painful energy, letting her expand left and right, up and down, embodying her freedom and confidence. I am happy to feel a shift of the pain, but also a confidence in my relationship with my body, an awareness of my holding onto others' conflicts, and an acceptance of the pain as a message. I leave with a curiosity as to what the next layer will be and the knowledge that I can let it go, whatever it is, and gradually move closer to my goal of a pain-free life.

—Olivia H.

Shadow

"People will do anything, no matter
how absurd, in order to avoid facing their own souls.
One does not become enlightened by imagining figures
of light, but by making the darkness conscious."

—C. G. Jung

What we call the Shadow is, perhaps, the most powerful protector of all. When there is something that we cannot accept in ourselves, we deny it even exists in ourselves, disowning it. We then project that quality or characteristic onto another and judge it in them.

Nonetheless, the Shadow is always following us around like a dragon's tail that is out of our awareness. And when we go into any metaphorically enclosed space, we create destruction, yet there is no possibility that we can become aware of how destructive we have been until we see the rubble.

Even then, what's most likely is that we'll hold someone(s) else responsible and accountable. Only when we are the only one who is consistently present when the destruction occurs may it begin to occur to us that the problem is not outside of ourselves, but that we are the unwitting destroyer. Or, as the saying goes, "We have met the enemy, and it is us."

The Shadow is not just made up of "negative" aspects of the self; it can be "positive" aspects also. If, for example, we can't own our own specialness, we will project that onto some other person and "judge" it in them by idealizing them. This can lead to craving and envy or simply an inability to own the gift in ourselves. Any comparison wed with judgmentalism is the basis for a shadow. In comparison with others, it can show up as an inferiority or superiority complex, judgmentalism about moral deficiency or virtue, anything that we can denigrate or idealize.

The more common version of Shadow is the negative one. It can reveal itself in one or both of two ways. First, and most insidiously, we can be judgmental of someone and think we are better than they are because we can't own some quality that we see in them. So, we experience them as fundamentally different from us, and we revile them for the difference.

Second, we can be judgmental because the action of the other person brings up some quality in us, and we find this quality in ourselves unacceptable. For example, another's action may force us to face our own helplessness, and we can't sit with that quality in ourselves. Another's action may make us face our own stupidity, even though the content of the other's stupidity is not the same as our own. Or, another's "lack of control" may ask us to face our own lack of control, though we are able to control ourselves in the area they are not able to control.

When we call someone deplorable instead of calling their actions deplorable, that is Shadow.

A simple example of the first version of Shadow is a person who gossips about everyone and everything. Then, when they are the subject of someone's gossip, they have extreme judgment about the person who shared about them, never recognizing that they do exactly the same thing to everyone all the time.

More extreme examples of this include someone who is profoundly judgmental of someone because of that other's judgmentalism, not recognizing and/or justifying their own judgmentalism. Or someone who is xenophobic, projecting their sense of inferiority because they are too afraid to experience it in themselves. Any "phobic" response to a person or people may qualify as this first type of "negative" Shadow. The man who preaches vehemently against homosexuals and then gets caught kissing another man is also an example of this.

An example of the second kind of negative Shadow may be the parent who is profoundly judgmental of and feels hatred for a pedophile. This is not only because pedophilia is about an adult who is hurting an innocent child but in addition because of the parent's own fear that they can't protect their child; they are unable to sit with their own helplessness and powerlessness about this. Or, a person who judges outsiders because of their fear that their way of life is threatened, and the person can't live with this fear.

To have this conversation about freeing ourselves from the power of Shadow, we must distinguish discernment from judgmentalism. Discernment invites us to maintain a centered perspective and to not get carried away by strong emotion. It presents us with an opportunity to make the right choices and to take positive actions. For example, a parent whose child is murdered may advocate for the murderer to be imprisoned because he or she is a danger to society, but that parent would not insist on vengeance via the "an eye for an eye" philosophy. We recognize that while this is easy to say in theory, it can be very hard in practice when something affects you deeply and personally. Moving to a place of discernment in all situations is a North Star that we can all aspire to, though it is very difficult to get to.

With this as introduction, let's go back to Nate and see how Shadow might have played out in his circumstance. In the situation where Nate continues to play out a version of his original role and behavior, he might become extremely judgmental of anyone who acts like they don't care or who gets depressed.

Working with Shadow

A very simple and powerful way to work with Shadow is called the finger-pointing exercise. Find someone or some group with whom you compare yourself in a judgmental fashion. In your mind's eye, start wagging your finger at them and going after them in the most lacerating, vicious, delicious way you can. Notice what sensation(s) arise as you are doing the practice.

Notice that when you point a finger at them, you're pointing three fingers back at yourself. Become the sensation(s) from the inside out, and then ask, "[Name of sensation], what have you come to share about how I am exactly like this person or group that I am comparing myself to and judging?" If you are brutally honest with yourself, it might become clear very quickly. You will also begin to see how you have played out in the world exactly what you are accusing them of. It can be very hard when you come to the realization that you are exactly like the person you feel so superior to. The same is true when you apply it in a situation where you feel inferior.

We have come a long way in this journey of understanding how our problems and reactivity can be forgotten choices to invite in obscuring protectors. We do this to keep our truer selves hidden and secure in reaction to something even worse than the presenting problem. It provides understanding for and a way to unravel an array of behaviors that would otherwise be very difficult to understand. Our hope is that it sheds some light on a challenging experience that you are facing and brings resolution and rediscovery of the truth of all of who you are, as well as the concomitant sense of aliveness that accompanies this. We hope the following exercise will give you a glimpse of the value of doing this kind of work.

EXERCISE

Think of a time that you have eaten for comfort. Most of us can probably find at least one time when we have done this. Many of us know this very well. Bring all your attention to "eating for comfort," scan your body, and notice any sensations that are there. Bring all your attention to the sensations to such a degree that you are becoming the sensations from the inside out. Then simply ask, "[Name of Sensations], what have you come to share about how eating for comfort protected me?" Be openly receptive to whatever the sensation(s) has come to share with you. You may find a narrative, or you may simply find the ways that comfort eating has protected you from difficult feelings and what those difficult feelings are, such as loneliness, boredom, emptiness, and so forth. With this information, the next time you reach to eat for comfort, before you put the piece of cake in your mouth, you may want to take a moment and ask, "Comfort Food, what have you come to protect me from?"

CHAPTER 11

The Enneagram of Personality: What Makes Us Tick

In this book so far, we have talked about how Life evolves through us and how what we experience as trauma is also Life's way of helping us grow and, through that growth, create more love. We have discussed different ways that we are traumatized in our life experience and ways to heal trauma, all in the service of reaching greater freedom.

Now, we are going to leave behind life experience and turn to Soul experience. Everything we have learned about life experience applies to Soul experience. There is one significant difference; there is only one trauma in Soul experience. This trauma is called the existential anxiety of non-existence. It is the most basic of all traumas and is intrinsic to being embodied. It creates the lens through which we perceive, understand, and react to all of Life and defend against this Soul trauma.

In this chapter we will explore these lenses, called our personalities, and the gifts and challenges that accompany them. To begin, we will name our different personalities which reveal how we act in the world and what motivates us. We will discover how we make meaning and where our attention naturally goes. Discovering more about ourselves opens another avenue through which we gain greater freedom, the freedom to respond from a place of choice as opposed to reacting automatically. We will do all this by learning about a system called the Enneagram.

In Chapter 12, we will show you how, in response to our one Soul trauma, the personality structures develop. We will go on to teach you how to work with this trauma by naming the underlying fears that accompany it for each of the personality structures, and how to release the hold these fears have on us so that we can truly live in greater freedom. We can then move from compulsive behavior to being able to live out the highest virtues and qualities of our personalities.

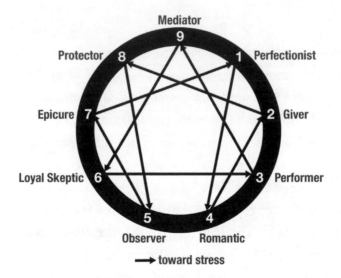

The word *Enneagram* is derived from the Greek words *enneas* meaning nine and *gramas* meaning points—literally nine points. This ancient system of understanding personality describes fundamental personality types, their core motivations (based on the avoidance of a core fear), and ways of relating in the world, each with its own gifts, natural limitations, and blind spots. This idea of nine personality types links it to the mysteries of many philosophical/religious traditions, and its psychological wisdom is consistent and compatible with modern personality theory. The system has much to teach us about ourselves.

When I, Joni, was first introduced to the Enneagram, I learned about my "point" and honestly felt nonplussed about what all the hype was about. My superficial review of the system missed the significance of all it offered. Not long after, my husband typed himself. Being married for nearly twenty-five years at the time, I thought that I knew all there was to know about this man, although I would admit that, as in most marriages, there were ways he acted at times that left me wanting to bang my head against the wall. After reading the twenty-five-page explanation of Enneagram Point Nine, new worlds of understanding opened up about who David is and why he acts the way he does. In that moment, reactivity had an opportunity to shift into understanding. I recall following him around the house after I read it, asking if this, that, and the other thing were true for him. The answer to all my questions was yes. I marveled at the understanding I gained that day, became hooked on this system, never looked back, and have been a devoted student of the Enneagram ever since.

By understanding our core motivations and underlying core fears, we are more able to begin to appreciate what drives our ways of being in the world. This begins to explain what feels like the inexplicable differences among us. Typically, our understanding is limited by our own frame of reference. When we begin to look at core motivations that drive our ways of being, we can open to much greater awareness and appreciation not only of ourselves but of others as well, and we can improve our interactions dramatically.

I will share one story about the usefulness of understanding core motivation before we move on to the nuts and bolts of this system.

I first introduced my daughter, now in her thirties, to the Enneagram when she was eight and in third grade. I had the opportunity to do it one morning when she and I were up early and the rest of the family slept. We were having special mother/daughter time, and I asked her what she would like for breakfast. "Blueberry pancakes! With lots of blueberries, Mommy!" she exclaimed. We went off to the kitchen where she sat at the counter, watching while I prepared and cooked the pancakes.

It was while she was eating and I cleaning up from the preparation that the opportunity to teach her about the Enneagram availed itself. I am what is known in Enneagram terms as an Eight, the Protector. Ale, my lovely daughter, is a Four, the Romantic. In general, an Eight's way of being is characterized by directness and is motivated by doing things in a way that assures a bottom-line result, while a Four's way is characterized by being special and is motivated by knowing and being sensitive to people's feelings. As we were chatting, I noticed a crumbled napkin in the trash with squished, partially uncooked pancake in it.

Hmmm, my first reaction was to say, "Ale, why did you throw out the pancakes? If they aren't cooked enough, you should tell me so I can make them how you like them." Bottom-line result! I stopped myself and thought about why my Enneagram Four daughter might not do what I considered the only reasonable thing to do if your mom gives you uncooked pancakes.

I thought of the situation from her perspective: Mom is trying to make me happy by making me my favorite breakfast. Mom isn't making me happy because she isn't cooking the pancakes enough. I can take care of and be sensitive to Mom by not letting her know that the pancakes aren't cooked; I'll eat what I can and throw the rest out without her seeing because that way Mom will feel good about what she is doing. (Because our responses are so automatic, we don't often realize what is going on until someone asks or we make a conscious choice to observe ourselves.)

What an opportunity for mother/daughter understanding! I showed Ale the crumbled napkin from the trash. She blushed. I told her I wasn't upset with her, but that we had a wonderful opportunity to better understand each other and how not understanding each other could lead to all sorts of bad feelings and hurt.

I asked her to explain to me why she put the uncooked pancakes in the trash. And just as I had suspected, she said something like, "Oh Mommy, you were being so nice to me making the blueberry pancakes just how I like them, and when they weren't cooked, I was sad because I didn't like them. I didn't want you to know I was sad because I wanted you to be happy and happy with me."

I told her the most important thing to me was for her to have those blueberry pancakes just the way she loved them. And, if that meant her telling me to do something different like cook them more or add more blueberries, or make them bigger or smaller, then that is exactly what I would want her to do. I went on to tell her that while she tried, from her perspective, to spare my feelings, she was actually doing something that if I didn't understand what was going on, would likely hurt my feelings. She really got it!

I went on to explain what might have happened if she had undercooked pancakes for me. I probably would have told her about it, thinking that I would be giving her the opportunity to give me the gift exactly as I wanted it which I would have assumed was exactly what she wanted me to do. She, on the other hand, would likely have experienced shame and me as ungrateful and have been hurt by my honesty.

In our new awareness, my precocious daughter and I giggled together like two people sharing a private joke. It actually was a pivotal moment in our relationship. Over the years, I have gotten better at recognizing my blind spots and slowing down my knee-jerk responses to take her into account, and we have gotten better at being able to acknowledge our differences and then in real time consider the other's perspective and adjust our way of being with each other accordingly, as a way to minimize misunderstanding and hurt. Of course, we aren't always perfect at it, but we have a foundation to understand the differences between us.

With that as an introduction, let's dive into the Enneagram system itself. We believe that, while we truly all are different, there are basically three kinds of people in this world. We call these people by names we can all understand: heart people, head people, and belly people. Each group has a core emotional and mental issue (more on that later). This is in alignment with the basic organizing principle of the Enneagram, which, as we said, states that there are nine personality types (different Enneagram authors have different names to capture the fundamentals of each type/point; however, the point number is consistent across all authors) arranged in three triads: the feeling (2, 3, 4), the thinking (5, 6, 7), and the sensing/doing (8, 9, 1). These triads correspond to the centers of perceptions (heart, head, and belly, respectively) through which we experience the world. While people use all three centers, each Enneagram type prefers to dominantly use one of them for perceiving and responding to Life.

We are learning all of this because what we are striving to discover is how to be fully present and not lose ourselves to our automatic ways of being. When we lose ourselves, we are not actually engaged with whatever Life is presenting us with in the moment. Instead, we rely on responses that are familiar and comfortable for us. The Enneagram teaches us about how we lose ourselves in these automatic ways. When applied to the centers, as we shall see, heart people lose themselves forward and out, seeking approval; head people lose themselves back and in seeking security; and belly people lose themselves up and diffuse (merging with their environments), reactively seeking identity.

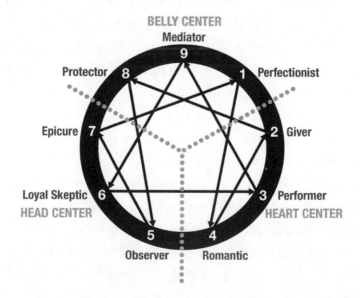

With this understanding, let's look at these three types/centers.

Heart People

Heart people are motivated by one fundamental question: Do you approve of me? What does it take to gain your approval? So, we can see, if someone is a heart person, their attention goes forward and out toward the other. They must create an image the other will positively respond to.

On a more surface level, heart people are not aware of what they are feeling. This is because authentic feelings may get in the way of the image they are creating and identifying with to gain the other's approval, and because their attention goes to the feelings of others in response to them. On a deeper level, heart people crave good feeling as an antidote to despair —the despair they would experience if they do not receive approval.

Head People

Head people are motivated by one fundamental question: Am I safe? In terms of relating to other people, the question is: Are you dangerous? The potential harm that is associated with this danger is that the other will demand too much or give too little. So, head people's attention goes backward and in, away from the other. They must scan for the danger the other may represent. In reaction to perceived danger, doubt is pervasive, including self-doubt. At the end of the day, it is better to be safe than sorry.

The feeling that head people must universally deal with is fear. If they can think through any situation, they can move away from danger, keeping fear at bay. On the surface level, they will perceive the danger as being external to them and their having to react to it. On a deeper level, the fear and doubt are within and create a core lens through which Life is interpreted.

Belly People

Belly people are not motivated by a question; they are motivated by circumstances. Lacking a sense of their own heart's desire, they find their identity by reacting to some external force. Because their attention moves to the external, they may not experience fear or craving. Lacking their own sense of who they are or what they desire, they merge and incorporate everything around them as a way of seeking identity. Therefore, their attention goes up and diffuses. While belly people can perceive what is happening and what must be done, this does not resolve the problem of knowing their own heart's desire.

The feeling that belly people must universally deal with is anger. It is ultimately anger at the self for not knowing one's true heart's desire and for not being able to act on it. As an antidote to this pain of self-forgetting, they keep themselves busy responding to the external aspects of life around them.

To review, there are three kinds of people: heart, head, and belly. Heart people lose themselves forward and out, creating an image to receive a response to attain a warm feeling to ward off despair. Head people lose themselves backward and in, believing that the world is a dangerous place that will demand too much and give too little. So, they feel a need to preserve what little they have in order to feel safe and to ward off fear. Belly people lose themselves up and diffuse, merging and incorporating everything around them as a way of seeking an identity in order not to experience the anger of forgetting their own hearts.

As we just explained, each of the centers has a dilemma that they are trying to manage. The three points of each center (totaling the nine Enneagram points) have different ways of resolving that dilemma. In each center (heart, head, belly), one point loses themselves forward and out, another back and in, and the third up and diffuse. We will discover that this direction explains how the person in each variation loses themselves with regard to their core emotional and mental issues.

HEART POINTS
(ENNEAGRAM POINTS 2, 3, 4)

Core Mental Issue: Image
Core Emotional Issue: Despair

Point 2, the Giver:
Externalization of Image and Despair

Givers lose themselves forward and out regarding despair and image. They look to the particular other to find out what image to portray to get that important other's approval. As long as they have that other's approval, they are invariably upbeat, even, in the classical sense, comic. In other words, the way to avoid despair is to actively deny it in themselves and to project it onto others and care for them. As long as the cared-for other is appreciative of the Giver, life is good.

Givers are people oriented and have a "we the people" approach to life. They like to be the power behind the throne. They focus on interpersonal experiences. They are cheerful and supportive. They know what people need and provide it for them. They are driven by emotional connection and can be so people-pleasing that they lose their own agendas. As a result, they find it very difficult to ask others for care, and therefore they can be manipulative as a way of getting their needs met. They are conflict averse. More than anything, they need to be needed and appreciated.

Gifts: helpful, caring, concerned, thoughtful, energetic

Challenges: can be manipulative, can be smothering, can be emotional, can give to get and then get angry if unappreciated

Point 3, the Performer: Identification with
Image and Denial of Despair

Performers lose themselves up and diffuse. They look to the general other to find the most apt image to gain approval through achieving success. Failure that would lead to despair is not an option. Vainly, they believe that who they are is the image they project. To avoid despair, they must deceive themselves that they have been dishonest. What we mean by this is that they deceive the world by creating and presenting an image, and then they deceive themselves that they have created this image.

Performers are people with a "can-do, fast-forward" attitude and often expect the same of others. They always seem to be in motion and making things happen. They are high achievers and high producers. They are optimistic and magnetic. They are often charismatic leaders. Failure does not exist for them. They create an appearance of success, believing reality will follow. They can be superficial, arrogant, and driven without reflection. They may not take others into account in their drive to achieve their own vision. They can want to succeed at any cost.

Gifts: hardworking, effective, positive, practical, efficient

Challenges: can be impatient, can have difficulty relaxing, can be superficial, can be insensitive about others' feelings

Point 4, the Romantic: Internalization of Image and Despair

Romantics lose themselves backward and in. They look inside for seeming authenticity, but it is not true authenticity. Instead, it is a unique image that discounts that which they are ashamed of. They then project it out to the world, implicitly demanding approval. Romantics constantly fight despair. Yet, no matter how much they compulsively move to grandiosity, self-denigration may never be far away. Romantics internalize despair and are therefore, in the classical sense, tragic.

Romantics are creative, inventive, think-outside-the-box kind of people. They tend to see the big picture. They are oriented toward elegance and authenticity. They are intense and reflective. They connect with others. Their personal feelings color everything. Rules don't apply to them. They can make people feel inadequate. They may have difficulty staying on task when feelings arise.

Gifts: sensitive, deep, intuitive, creative, passionate

Challenges: can be self-absorbed, can be dramatic, can be dissatisfied
with self and others, can long for what is missing, can feel like a
misfit

HEAD POINTS
(ENNEAGRAM POINTS 5, 6, 7)

Core Mental Issue: Paranoia or Doubt
Core Emotional Issue: Fear

Point 5, the Observer:
Internalization of Doubt and Fear

Observers lose themselves backward and in reaction to doubt and
fear. They limit what they need so they will not have to ask for anything.
When asked for anything, whether it be material, knowledge, or time, they
go inside and do an inventory of how much resource they have before
responding. In the face of fear, they move back to a place of protection,
literally or energetically, so that they are out of harm's way. Nonetheless,
the doubt and fear are still internalized and are experienced as deficiency
or insufficiency with associated anxiety.

Observers are wise, self-sufficient people. They tend to be compart-
mentalized thinkers. They are analytical, and they absorb facts and details,
then formulate new perspectives. Their attention goes to ideas over people.
They are able to not get pulled into the emotions of a situation. They fear
losing their energy and being drained. They can be isolated, distant, and
withholding, and others can find it difficult to connect with them. They
can be judgmental around a display of emotions. They protect themselves
and feel safe by hoarding.

Gifts: thoughtful, dependable, even-tempered, curious, exacting, per-
ceptive, nonmaterialistic

Challenges: can be standoffish and unapproachable, can be private to a fault, can lack consideration of others' feelings, can be unable to make decisions without getting more information

Point 6, the Loyal Skeptic: Identification with Doubt and Denial of Fear

Loyal Skeptics lose themselves up and diffuse in reaction to doubt and fear. It's as if the doubt makes them dissociative, in that they may doubt the world and then question their own doubt, causing them to doubt themselves. Disidentifying with the fact that they create their own fear, they experience it as a reaction to potentially threatening external things. Not able to get away from fear, they may fight, flee, or freeze.

Loyal Skeptic are team players. They see things that can go wrong. They are loyal and love who you are, not your image. They are responsible and focused. They support the underdog. They are willing to question authority. They are contrarians. They can be oppositional, pessimistic, and paralyzed by doubt of the world and self; others may find them negative and a downer.

Gifts: reliable, careful, trustworthy, dedicated, considerate

Challenges: can be ambivalent, can procrastinate, can feel challenged by authority, can see all that is wrong but not what is right in a situation

Point 7, the Epicure: Externalization of Doubt and Fear

Epicures lose themselves forward and out in reaction to doubt and fear. Nothing bad can happen; every problem is just an opportunity. Life is to be filled with pleasant options so as not to limit the self. In fact, the only fearful thing is to be limited because limitation can lead to a restriction of filling oneself up with what is best.

Epicures are brainstormers and synthesizers. They are creative and see how things fit together in a new way. They are visionary. They prefer to have multiple pleasant options. They thrive in multitasking environments. They can get projects started but need support to follow through because they can perceive the follow-through as boring and therefore painful. They tend to break down hierarchies. Easily distracted, Epicures hate being bored and feeling trapped. They can get caught up in the "Everything is a learning opportunity" momentum, leading to rationalization. They can exhibit lack of commitment, responsibility, and empathy.

Gifts: enthusiastic, playful, inventive, optimistic, big-picture thinkers

Challenges: can get easily bored, can feel trapped, can exhibit lack of commitment, responsibility, and empathy

BELLY POINTS (ENNEAGRAM POINTS 8, 9, 1)

Core Mental Issue: Self-Forgetting
Core Emotional Issue: Anger

Point 8, the Protector: The Externalization of Self-Forgetting and Anger

Protectors lose themselves forward and out in reaction to self-forgetting and anger. They focus on excess and getting what they sense they want in the world as a substitution for knowing their heart's desire. Unaware that they are actually angry for forgetting themselves, they are reactively angry in life and express it openly with people, often in direct, outspoken ways.

Protectors are honest, straightforward, and natural leaders. They have larger-than-life energy for projects personally perceived as important. They will stand up and move against powerful opposition in the service of getting the job done. Their focus is on justice. They are excellent team players if they respect team members and/or feel that they legitimately need protection. They are practical, believing that the end justifies the means. They are willing to meet conflict head-on and are prone to outbursts of anger. They can be impulsive, and people can experience them as insensitive to their feelings, and sometimes punitive.

Gifts: strong, resourceful, tenacious, straightforward, truthful

Challenges: can often be intimidating, can be impulsive, can be vin-
dictive, can be overpowering, can be insensitive

Point 9, the Mediator:
The Identification with Self-Forgetting
and the Denial of Anger

Mediators lose themselves up and diffuse in reaction to self-forgetting
and anger. They merge with others as a substitution for knowing themselves and their own needs. Having forgotten themselves, disidentifying
with their own anger, they are visions of harmony, peace, and acceptance.
A mediator is often the quintessential "nice guy."

Mediators are kind, even, and display goodwill. They acknowledge,
appreciate, and mediate all points of view. They find commonalities. They
are very productive within a structure. They are great team players and are
willing to do any task. They care little about the limelight and are humble.
They take on others' points of views as their own. They space out easily.
These "lost children" can feel and act as though they don't matter. Others
can find their lack of initiative and their inability or unwillingness to share
their point of view as problematic.

Gifts: caring, adaptive, gentle, easygoing, attentive

Challenges: can lose priorities and get lost in non-essential tasks, can
be stubborn in a passive-aggressive manner, can lack vision and
passion, can be dominated by a drive for comfort

Point 1, the Perfectionist: The Internalization
of Self-Forgetting and Anger

Perfectionists lose themselves back and in reaction to self-forgetting
and anger. They focus on living up to a righteous, ethical point of view
based on taking correct action in the world. They substitute rightness for
knowing and experiencing their own needs. This leads to an internalized

anger at the self. This anger can leak out self-righteously toward others.

Perfectionists are visionaries, particularly around high standards and goal achievement. They are organized, efficient, and detail oriented. They get the job done on time with excellence. They believe in self-improvement and are therefore self-critical. They are clear communicators. Their motto is to work first and play second. They can get lost in the details of their visions and miss the big picture. For them, life is about doing things right.

> **Gifts:** sensible, responsible, self-reliant, hardworking, precise, dependable

> **Challenges:** can be judgmental, can be critical, can be harsh, can be nitpicky, can be difficult to challenge

Given that there are nearly 8 billion people in the world, how can nine ways of being account for all the differences among us? You may have read the above and felt that you resonated with several of the Enneagram points and can't land on just one. The Enneagram is a fluid model that accommodates all of our human differences as well as the nonstatic nature of our human personality. Each point on the diagram is only a partial representation of a person's type. Each individual's personality is actually a unique combination of all of the points, with primary motivators reflecting their fundamental personality point and some degree of the particular aspects of adjacent points, which are called *wings*. Additionally, while retaining our own fundamental personality point, when we feel secure, we tend to move in a consistent direction to another point called the secure point. When experiencing stress, we tend to move in a consistent direction to our stress point. The relationship of movements to other points is illustrated on the diagram.

As an example, if I am an Enneagram Point 8, the Protector, I can have aspects to my personality of Point 7, the Epicure, and Point 9, the Mediator. Point 7 will contribute a fun-loving optimism while Point 9 will contribute a softness and kindness. Different Enneagram Point 8s will have different amounts of those adjacent points, which will affect their way of being in the world and what they look like to others. In addition, when I am stressed, I will move to Point 5, the Observer, pulling back and becoming more thoughtful and quieter. In security, when things are going well in my life, I will naturally gravitate to Enneagram Point 2, the Giver, and become more magnanimous. So, just for Point 8 alone, there are practically an infinite number of weighted combinations of the three Points 7, 8, 9 to account for the many differences seen in different Point 8s with movement, in any given moment, to stress and secure points adding to those differences.

Subtypes

Subtypes are our most fundamental instinctual drives. Enneagram theory lists three subtypes or drives: security, connection, and belonging. While they are intrinsically part of the human condition, they also have a compulsive quality. Like our personalities, they protect us from the core fears of basic insecurity, disconnection, and not belonging. While each of us has all these fears, one predominates in each of us. Our *need* to be secure, our *need* to connect, and our *need* to belong keeps us from feeling the internal anxiety of insecurity, lack of connection, and lack of belonging. This allows us to bring our attention outside of ourselves as opposed to within. No matter how much we have, we ultimately feel insecure; no matter how good our relationships, we ultimately feel alone; and no matter how much we participate, we ultimately feel like we don't belong.

There are two ways to recognize subtypes. The first way is to imagine yourself at a party and notice where your primary focus of attention goes. If you are a securing subtype, called *self-preserving* in this system, you are likely to seek the food, something to drink, and a place to sit or stand. You're likely to search out how to make yourself feel safe and comfortable there, taking your physical needs and the needs of others into account. If you are a connecting subtype, called *sexual* in this system (even though it is not about sex per se) you are likely to look for someone at the party with whom you can connect and have a "meaningful" experience, often to the exclusion of others. If you are a belonging subtype, called *social* in this system, you will very likely make yourself part of the group, act inclusively, and interrupt your conversation with one person to be sure the person who joins you isn't left out.

The second way to recognize subtype is by following energy as a way of knowing. A self-preserving subtype's energy goes back and in to secure its own needs and the needs of others who are significant through incorporation. A sexual subtype's energy lasers forward and out through the eyes to connect with a particular other. Finally, a social subtype's energy goes up and diffuses to participate with the whole.

As a consequence of subtype, there are three variations of each personality type, totaling twenty-seven in all, each of which looks somewhat different than the other.

Knowing a person's Enneagram point of view, center, and subtype helps us to understand how they are likely to relate to the world. We gain more awareness of where they focus their attention and what is truly important to them. It follows that it also gives us nuanced information about how they are likely to be in relationship. With great accuracy, we are able to predict the satisfactions and challenges that typically arise for each Enneagram pairing. For example, if a couple is getting engaged, and one is a sexual subtype and the other a social subtype, they are likely to have vastly different views on the "perfect" engagement. The sexual subtype might imagine a weekend away, just the two of them alone on a beach when the proposal happens. Only after sharing the moment would they consider calling families. The social subtype may conjure up the idea of the proposal happening at a party where everyone could celebrate together.

More than any tool we have encountered, the Enneagram helps us to learn to be truly empathic toward others and their way in the world while keeping our own perspective. It's a way of getting to know ourselves and others from the inside out.

It's a system that helps us understand and appreciate our differences, move to a place of receptivity versus reactivity, and open to our gifts, both individually and collectively.

Emotional maturity significantly increases our access to our gifts and strengths, while more limited emotional development tends to increase reactivity and produce destructive rather than constructive behaviors (e.g., Franklin Delano Roosevelt and Saddam Hussein were both Point 8s— Protectors). Emotional maturity is developed by being able to allow our fears as opposed to compulsively compensate for them.

> *I appreciate the integration of the wisdom of the Enneagram and find pleasure in knowing my type and observing the behaviors that come with the territory. Moments of crystal-clear truth emerge and replace feelings of fear, worry, and anxiety. I continue to learn from and to transform my experience of traumatic loss.*
>
> —Gloria

Discovering Your Type

Before we move on, let's stop and take a minute to let you assess what your Enneagram type is. (For middle-aged and older readers, sometimes it's easier to look back at how you acted in your twenties.) The best way to do that is to follow the maps in this chapter by first discerning what center most resonates with you about your focus of attention in the world. When you are really honest with yourself, is your primary motivation to seek approval (heart), to keep yourself safe (head), or to be responsible (belly)?

If you are a heart point, is the primary way you try to get people to like you through:

a) Taking care of their needs so you will be indispensable to them (Point 2)?

b) Performing and being successful so you get recognition and applause (Point 3)?

c) Being unique so people will think you are special (Point 4)?

If you are a head point, is the primary way you stay safe through:

a) Being self-sufficient and minimizing your needs (Point 5)?

b) Anticipating all the bad things that can happen and taking a "yes, but" point of view (Point 6)?

c) Making sure you keep yourself occupied with pleasant options so you don't feel the pain in life (Point 7)?

If you are a belly point, is the primary way you respond through:

a) Taking charge, protecting those you care about, and hierarchically knowing what is called for in a situation (Point 8)?

b) Seeking harmony and comfort and going with the flow (Point 9)?

c) Knowing and doing the right thing because that is the right thing to do (Point 1)?

Finally, try to determine your subtype. Do you primarily focus on security around material things like food, shelter, and money (self-preservation)? Do you primarily want and need to have a relationship where you can intensely connect (sexual)? Does belonging and participating seem essential to a happy life (social)? The subtypes are stacked—primary, secondary, and tertiary—adding up to 100 percent. Some people's weightings are more balanced while others are more extreme.

The invitation in learning your Enneagram point is so that you can begin to understand the lens through which you see Life, rather than simply looking through that lens with unawareness. By doing this, you can begin to appreciate the limitation and the gifts of your particular lens, and begin the process of freeing yourself from automatically reacting.

To come full circle from where we started in this chapter, perhaps the most powerful application of the Enneagram is using it as a tool for spiritual growth. The Enneagram suggests that our personalities (and even our deepest ways of perceiving and our deepest instinctual drives) are, in part, compulsions that serve as protections from experiencing our deepest fears about ourselves. It reveals what these fears are. When we are able to become aware of, allow, and accept these deepest fears about ourselves, we're able to realize and touch into our Essence (the ultimate, fundamental, pure aspect of our being)—the everything. In the following chapter, we will teach you a practice to work with these fears, lessening the grip of your personality and bringing you closer to Essence. In Essence, we know what is true for us, we know what we truly desire, and we know the best way to make it happen.

CHAPTER 12

Personality as a Protection

What is the point of understanding personality as a protection? Having just identified our Enneagram type and learned about our core mental and emotional issues as well as the gifts and limitations of our personalities, we are now going to explore the idea that our personalities are just compulsive reactions to an underlying core fear. Most of us are not aware of what these fears are, and the attributes of our personality can give us hints as to the fears that lie beneath. When we do identify that fear, fully allow and accept it, its hold on us diminishes, and we are freer to live in the full richness of all of who we are.

Let's start with a story that may give you some idea what this chapter is about and how it can benefit you. Early in my Enneagram training, I, Andy, and a friend, who is an Enneagram Point 4, a Romantic, went to an Enneagram workshop taught by one of the most well-regarded teachers in the field. The workshop had a panel format, which meant that a few of each of the nine types, who considered themselves to have perspective on their type, would go up and share about themselves to the group.

My friend was one of the students who was on the Type 4 panel. When he started to talk about being a Four, he was intense and dramatic, while telling people he had worked hard and overcome this in his personality. He shared that he felt he lived with a sense of equanimity which is the North Star for this point. (In Enneagram language, this is called the virtue of Type 4.) His sharing revealed anything but achieving what he claimed.

A fellow participant came up to him after the panel and said that it seemed to her that his presentation belied his capacity to be free of his compulsions, that it seemed to her that he was showing us what it was like when a Type 4 needed to be special and dramatic. As she was loudly saying this to him, out of the corner of his eye he could see people, including the teacher, nodding their head in agreement.

He felt extremely ashamed (a likely Type 4 response) because he believed he had made such a fool of himself in front of all his peers and teacher. The core fear of Type 4 is about being defective, and the experience he just had touched him into this. He wanted to find the nearest rock he could hide under and not come out.

Returning to the room we shared, he went on for quite some time while licking his wounds about how awful he was and how everyone was laughing at him. I commiserated with him about how much pain he was in and shared how, but for the grace of God, I could've been in the same situation up in front of the group, revealing my fixations. I suggested we do a practice to help him get through how he was feeling in the moment.

I invited him just to fully allow and bring all his attention to the shame he felt about being so defective and that he would be shunned because of what he had done. I asked him to notice what was happening in the body and just choose to bring all his awareness to whatever discomfort was there, become it, and let it share. As he did this and allowed all the difficult feelings from the experience he had just had and the sense of defectiveness that fed those feelings, he began to lacerate himself even more, remembering all the times he had "made a fool of himself" and felt so ashamed. As he was giving full expression to these difficult feelings, something counterintuitive happened. He noticed that he started to calm down, the sensation was dissipating, and his body began to relax. He then said, "It's hard for me to believe this, but what just happened on the panel doesn't feel like that big a deal anymore. Maybe I am beginning to get a sense of equanimity." And in that moment, a new possibility was born.

The Point of It All: Freedom

Let's go back to basics and remember what this book is about and what's in it for you. In a word, *freedom*. The invitation of this book is to remember who we truly are so that we are free to be fully present in every moment: free to be omniscient, meaning all-knowing and entirely open minded; free to be omnipotent, meaning all-powerful, which in this case means to be fully engaged and know that everything is possible and then ultimately, to be engaged in the creative process of bringing it to Life; free to be omnibenevolent, meaning all-loving and entirely open hearted.

Most of us, most of the time, don't aspire to reach the summit of freedom. Nonetheless, if we start the journey, we begin to notice that we are freer and less living on automatic; more fully present and less in trance, so to speak. And typically, when we are living on automatic, eventually it comes to be unsatisfying, even if it was previously something on which we based our identity. Yet when we are early in our lives, we don't typically realize we are living on automatic. We just think we are living.

Where We Begin

Given what we have said above, most of us live lives of relative compulsion based on avoidance of an underlying fear. Let's go back to the Enneagram to understand what this means. If I have the structure of Point 1, Perfectionist, I will know that there is a right way to live life, and that everybody ought to live life by the same rules and principles that I do, except that I may have a principle that says that everybody should be allowed a little bit to be who they are; but, of course, even that would be a rule.

Early in my life, I would wonder why everybody doesn't understand the world the way I do. Isn't it clear to them that there is the right way to live?! Isn't it clear that work ought to always come before pleasure? It's perhaps only later in life that I may begin to question this. Perhaps enough people have called me a stick-in-the-mud or too tight or judgmental or something. In the beginning, I might wonder, *Don't they understand that I'm a good, nice person?* But if enough people say this to me, I may begin to wonder if it may have something to do with me. I may begin to think that "all work and no play makes Jack a dull boy."

Even if I begin to come to the realization that my way of being may be limited, I find, perhaps a little bit to my chagrin, that I can't help myself. I can't stop making lists. I can't ever let myself relax before everything is done. Why do I do this? To avoid a core fear of *I am bad*. How can I begin to change? Stay with us.

Every point has its own version of this story and its accompanying fear. If I'm a Giver, I have to put other people first and be pleasing, even when it causes me to deny my own needs and then become resentful because I have a fear of being unworthy. If I'm a Performer, I have to keep succeeding no matter what, even when it causes me to push so hard that I never relax and just be because I have a fear of being a failure. If I'm a Romantic, I have to compulsively be special, even when I see how that compulsion can make me miserable because I have a fear of being defective. If I'm an Observer, I have to be self-sufficient, even when I can see that it limits me and keeps me from reaching out in a loving way because I have a fear of being insufficient. If I'm a Loyal Skeptic, I have to be secure, even when I realize that my angst might be driving myself and everyone around me crazy because I have a fear of being a nobody. If I'm an Epicure, I have to have the most pleasant, exciting experience, even if it means that I break commitments and leave the people around me hanging because I have a fear of being unfulfillable. If I'm a Protector, I have to be the one who's in control, even when I realize that I am running other people's lives at my own expense because I have a fear of being impotent. If I'm a Mediator, I have to create harmony, even if it means I will put up with anything because I have a fear of being unlovable.

Requirements for Change

Admittedly, most of these problems concerning compulsions do mellow with time. Either we have a crisis that forces us to reassess, or we just get tired. Nonetheless, even if it is not as compelling, it's still as compulsive, and we still can't stop. The question is, why can't I change?

The reason we have such a difficult time changing is because typically the way we live and the things we do, we do compulsively. We are not behaving these ways just because they are "who we are." We are behaving this way to protect us, as we said earlier, from experiencing a fear we have about ourselves.

How did all this come to be? Remember what is foundational. We say that we lose our freedom when there's something that can't be taken in stride. Until this point, we have talked about what can't be handled in the world of life experience. We've discovered that when something can't be handled, we lose our perspective, and instead of remembering the experience and being identified with the holding witness, we identify with the one who is not able to handle the experience and the way they protect themselves in an attempt never to have to experience it again.

We are now going to take the same foundation and move it up a level from the world of matter and life experience to the world of Soul and the experience of embodiment. Embodiment is when we individuate from Source. On one level, this is a gift because we get to experience all the delicious sensual joys of being in a body. On another level, it is intrinsically traumatic, leading to the illusion of separation and limitation. Once we identify with being separate and limited, our sense of aliveness gets associated with and even dependent on maintaining that sense of separateness. Remembering who we truly are, which is everything, gets associated with nonexistence. The idea of nonexistence brings a sense of terror and an incapacity to even open to the possibility of re-membering and being who we truly are, the everything. Essentially, we all know something about nonexistence because we can relate to the fear of death of the physical body.

We're going to make a claim that may be startling for many of you—that whatever it is that you're most afraid to admit about yourself is the doorway to your Essential Self, the one who in everyday life is free to experience all of Life in whatever form it comes to them with a total sense of peace and acceptance, just being able to say, "yes." In actuality, the Essential Self is to be all of Life, which to the personality feels like nonexistence. As our teacher once said in an inscrutable way that she didn't explain, "The way to Essence is through the personality."

The Theory

So let's revisit what happens. We start by being everything. When we are created, we become something that is in God's image, meaning that God still exists and resides within us, yet we no longer remember our origin. Because of this, when we contemplate the journey of becoming who we truly are, that is, everything, then everything that we compulsively identify with disappears, with the consequent profound and total loss of self.

Looking at it from the point of view of the beings that are created, becoming who you truly are (the everything) is not liberation—it's annihilation. If you were a raindrop and you are being gravitationally pulled into an ocean, you might do everything you could to try to stop the forces of gravity because the second you hit the ocean, you might believe that you would cease to exist as that with which you identify—being the drop.

Instead of remembering and realizing who you truly are (the ocean and everything else), you would fully identify with the limited form (the drop) and experience who you truly are as death because, from the perspective of the drop, you would cease to exist, and it would be like you never existed.

So we choose to protect the true self from the feared total annihilation by identifying with "I." This identification moves us away from who we truly are which is Life itself. Because this limitation is experienced as a trauma, as is true with all traumas, we take on limiting beliefs which we call limited negative identities. From the perspective of "I," this limited negative identity is something we want to stay away from because it is the only barrier that protects from annihilation. We all can relate to wanting to get as far away as possible from something we think will consume us. To create the distance from the limited negative identity (for the Perfectionist, I am bad), we create a limited positive identity (for the Perfectionist, I am good), which defines our personality.

For each of us, our core fear continually pokes at us if we slow down and listen. It is why we generally don't slow down to the degree that is required to hear it. Instead, we do what we do —the "doing" having a different flavor for each of the Enneagram points.

If we did slow down enough, we might hear the following from the core fear in the haughtiest of voices: *Do you think you can get away from me?! Don't be ridiculous! You've been trying to get away from me for your whole life, and I'm still here. I've been here from the very beginning, I'm here now, and I will always be here. And you can run, but you can't hide. You can hate me, curse me, deny me, pretend I don't exist. And at the end of the day, I will always be here, and there's one thing I can assure you of which is that I will never leave, and you can never get rid of me, get me to go, no matter how hard you try! No matter what you do!*

Now we'll share with you what traditionally Source/God is thought to share with us in the most loving of voices: *I promise, no matter what you do, I will always be with you. I've been here from the very beginning, I'm here now, and I will always be here. You can try to run away from Me, and you can't hide. You can hate Me, you can curse Me, you can deny Me, and you can even pretend I don't exist. It doesn't matter what you do, I promise I will never abandon you, and I will always be with you. You can count on that.*

As you can see, that which we are most afraid to admit about ourselves and Source say exactly the same thing! It's just that we have called Source by the wrong name and have spent our whole life trying to get away. Yet, Source, in Its love, keeps calling us back. It's like the gravitational pull of a black hole that is so much bigger than us. And what is gravity if not two things being brought together, or, to put it differently, Love? This is a gift from Life to our Souls in that it is a constant reminder of the fullness of Life that is available to us if we do something counterintuitive and go into it. When we choose to let go and go in, we discover that our anxiety was misplaced; we discover Essence.

The Benefits for Each Point

What is the result of no longer being compelled by your core fear? Let's look at it for each personality type.

If you are a Perfectionist (Point 1), you will find that you get to keep your vision and principles, and you will come to know that it is not your job to perfect Life. You'll discover that Life is perfect just the way it is, including the changes that will naturally happen if you don't get in the way with the need to be perfectionistic and the worry that accompanies this. You will gain a sense of serenity and realize that you are doing your part in service to the evolution of Life.

If you are a Giver (Point 2), you will find that you still are extraordinary in terms of knowing and taking care of the needs of others. You just will no longer have to compulsively take care of these needs so that others will need you, so that you will get a sense of being worthwhile. You'll be able to give altruistically, from a place of freedom and humility, because your basic sense of worthiness will be internal and, even more, because your sense of identity is not dependent on others needing to depend on you. Miraculously, it is okay to have your own needs and to get them cared for by others.

If you are a Performer (Point 3), you will still be able to do and create things. You will no longer be doing it, in part, in order to feel like a success in the service of getting the applause of others. You will have a hope that if you were your true self and not your image, people would still accept and love you.

If you are a Romantic (Point 4), you will still be sensitive, creative, and oriented toward the deepest aspects of Life. You will no longer compulsively create a special image to gain people's attention. Your life will have a sense of equanimity over dissatisfaction with how normal your life is: you will not compare yourself to others from a sense of lack. You will not be self-absorbed and will transform egocentric longing into life-enhancing creation of beauty.

If you are an Observer (Point 5), you will still be self-sufficient, able to observe without being pulled by emotions, and able to gather all the information necessary to gain understanding and make the best choices. You will no longer compulsively have to gather every bit of information and need to build a wall around yourself; while you may be a rock, you will not have to be an island. No longer afraid of Life demanding too much or providing too little, you will move from simply gaining knowledge to having wisdom, from isolation to being engaged and empowered, and from withdrawing to experiencing and expressing your feelings, including vulnerable feelings of love.

If you are a Loyal Skeptic (Point 6), you will still be able to see and prepare for all the bad things that may happen, be able to take contrarian points of view so that all perspectives, including your own, will be considered, and be someone who is seen as trustworthy and reliable. You will no longer compulsively need to agonize over decisions, being plagued with the angst of doubt. You will have the courage and faith to face your fears and the discernment to know when Life is truly dangerous or when it's just your projection.

If you are an Epicure (Point 7), you will still know how to plan and have the best pleasant options for yourself and for those around you. You will still be able to be a synthetic, big-picture thinker and wonderful brainstormer and visionary entrepreneur. You will no longer compulsively be in a place of craving to have one good experience after another to the point of exhaustion. You will be able to make a commitment and keep it when Life calls for it. You won't participate in childish pranks or fraudulently take advantage of "a sucker that is born every minute." You will get to keep your childlike wonder and mature.

If you are a Protector (Point 8), you will still know how to be a natural leader, know how to make things happen, and understand hierarchy and how to apply it in all situations. You will no longer compulsively need to avoid a sense of weakness and vulnerability and know that sometimes weakness is true strength and vulnerability is the way not to deny the truth of your heartfelt inner experience. You will still be able to speak the truth and maintain an innocent sense of wonder.

If you are a Mediator (Point 9), you will still be able to viscerally know other people's perspectives, go with the flow, and keep harmony and peace. You will no longer have to do these things compulsively so that when Life calls for you to find what you desire and speak it, to take initiative, to be willing to have a conflict, you will not disappear. You will know the truth of your own heart as well as the truth of everybody else's. You will be able to act on priorities and not dissipate your energy on distractions.

A Call to Action

As you read what we are presenting, we invite you to consider what may be underlying your personality. You might start to do this by asking, *What am I most afraid to admit about myself? Is there anything even deeper than that? How do I protect myself from ever having to experience these fears?* The discovery of and resonance with these fears takes some work to get to. Believe us when we tell you it's worth the effort.

As you begin to ask these questions, you may notice that while the protection of your personality makes you feel comfortable, sometimes the fears may start to come up and the personality may have to work harder to keep them at bay. It is not for no reason that we spend so much energy trying to avoid these fears, believing all the time it is just who we are.

The end game here is to be able to enjoy and choose to share with the world all the gifts of your personality while minimizing the less desirable aspects of who we are. You will get to use your gifts in a freer, less ego-centric, more in-service-to-Life way. And in this way, life becomes more intrinsically satisfying.

Core Fears and the Enneagram: An Overview

The model we've found to be most efficient and elegant for identifying, understanding, and transforming our core fears is the Enneagram, which we taught you about in the previous chapter and talked about above.

To review, the basic organizing principle of this model is that nine personality points of view are arranged in three triads: the feeling (2, 3, 4), the thinking (5, 6, 7), and the sensing (8, 9, 1) triads that correspond to the centers of perceptions (heart, head, and belly) through which we experience the world. The nine types are further characterized by subtype or their most fundamental instinctual drive to either be secure, connected, or belong.

The Four Levels of Working

The Enneagram teaches us that we are afraid that who we are is the limited negative identities we referred to earlier. These identities come on four different levels: the level of personality (nine Enneagram points), the level of center (three centers: heart, head, belly), the level of subtype (three subtypes: self-preserving, sexual, social), and finally, the level of nonexistence itself.

When working with the trauma that arises out of embodiment and the four levels of associated fears, we call this "working with *Embodiment Identity*." Most typically, we begin working on the level of personality. For our purposes, we are only going to work with the level of personality in this book.

Nine Personalities

To review, each personality has a limited negative view of itself and the world, based on its core fear. As we talked about earlier, for example, the person whose core fear on the level of personality is *I am bad* will compulsively identify with *I am good, and I am a Perfectionist.* That person will not be able to experience their true goodness, their perfection, because in part they use their goodness/perfection as a way of compulsively compensating for their core fear of *I am bad.*

We substitute a particular quality (for example, *goodness*) for our ground of being (which is *is-ness,* or *I am*). In other words, we believe *I am good, therefore I am* rather than *I am, therefore I am good, bad, and everything else in the universe.* If we did something counterintuitive and went into the core fear, which we call, in this case, *I am bad,* we would find it is the doorway to the higher aspects of self. Once we have gone through this doorway and have freedom from the compulsion of our personality, we can use this as a doorway to the ultimate freedom of "no self"—Essence.

The following chart lists the nine personalities, their core fear, and the counterbalancing positive view that gives rise to the personality. Notice how the counterbalancing positive view can give rise to the names of each personality.

PERSONALITY–CORE FEARS		
PERSONALITY TYPE	LIMITED NEGATIVE VIEW (CORE FEAR)	COUNTERBALANCING POSITIVE VIEW (OBSCURING IDENTITY)
	I am:	**I am:**
1. Perfectionist	Bad	Good
2. Giver	Unworthy of existing	Worthy of existing
3. Performer	Failure	Success

PERSONALITY–CORE FEARS		
4. Romantic	Ordinary/Defective	Special
5. Observer	Insufficiency	Self-sufficient
6. Loyal Skeptic	Nobody	Somebody
7. Epicure	Unfulfillability	Fulfilled
8. Protector	Powerlessness/Controlled	Powerful/In control
9. Mediator	Chaos/Unloveability	Peace/Love

Compensations

Because it's so uncomfortable to experience our core fears, we do things in our lives that support us in getting away and staying away from them. There are things we tell ourselves about ourselves. They are primarily the positive counterbalancing view of our personalities, outlined in the table above. In addition, we use other people. We can seduce them into supporting this positive view of ourselves by getting them to tell us we are good, worthy, successful, and so on. We might busy ourselves with others, too, as a way to not feel the fear. On one level, because we are using people to protect us from our fears, we never get to be truly intimate with them.

We may keep ourselves active as a way not to feel the fear. Sometimes, even things that feel very negative in our lives may act as a protection. While most of us can understand, as painful as it is, how addictions can serve to protect us from having to experience a fear, as crazy as it sounds, even illnesses can provide the same kind of protection. As with all the other compensations, they try to serve us by protecting us from experiencing anxiety while simultaneously inviting us into that very anxiety. Sometimes, these avoidances take on a life of their own and are the doorway into finding the core fear. When the avoidance is the doorway in, we call it an Archetypal

Identity, because the avoidance has taken on archetypal proportions.

As an example, a chronic illness, like fibromyalgia, on one level, may serve us by diverting our attention away from our core fear. If you are an Enneagram Point 2 with a core fear of, "I am unworthy," then the illness may let you accept help from others, which typically would be very difficult to do because your sense of worthiness is based on taking care of others' needs while not having your own (you would see that as being needy). Yet the illness, at the same time, profoundly limits your capacity to live your life. It is important to note that we are not saying that resolving the relationship between your core fear and the illness will necessarily make either the illness or the core fear go away. What we are saying is that working with the hook that binds the two may allow you to be more at peace with the situation or allow your body to access its innate healing power to shift the illness toward greater health.

The Essence Process:
Lessen the Grip of Your Core Fears

The Essence Process is quite simple. We begin by becoming aware of, allowing, bringing all of our attention to and accepting the fear we are most afraid to experience about ourselves. After identifying and experiencing this fear, we are invited to name all the ways that we compensate for it, all the time feeling what is happening in the body. We then invite you to realize that, while we have this fear, and we spend a great deal of time and energy compensating for it, it is not who we are. If it truly is who we are, we cannot witness it. Because we are witnessing it and identifying with the witness that is choosing to witness it, we know that from that perspective, it is outside of ourselves. It is just one more experience, like looking at a chair. (The only difference is that we've previously given this experience far more power.) Therefore, we then use our consciousness to bring the fear outside ourselves and to externalize it, including all the sensations that arise in the body. (We can more easily do this when we realize it is energy just like us and everything else in the universe.) Once we bring this energy outside ourselves, we *expand* in all six directions simultaneously. (We do this by imagining that we can burst out of our body in all directions at the same time.) We do this to be and experience being the one consciousness which, in fact, we already are.

Finally, we reintegrate the energy we used to call the fear we were most afraid to experience by treating it, not as something that we hate, but as a guide whose wisdom we seek and honor and to which we give gratitude, respect, and love. We can do this either by recreating the energy that used to be our core fear or just speaking to it as part of the everything and asking it, *What is your greatest hope for me?* The answers that come can truly be extraordinary. When we discover that we are already that greatest hope, either the energy fully dissolves or turns alchemically into some extraordinary gift that we can keep with us like a promise and a friend.

HERE'S HOW TO DO IT STEP BY STEP:

1. **Begin by naming what you are most afraid of or ashamed to admit about yourself.** You can do this by using the Core Fears Chart above and see what resonates with you, or alternatively by muscle testing the chart. You can name it for yourself in your own words by checking in with yourself. If you are naming it yourself, keep digging by asking yourself if there is anything worse than what you have just said, until you get to a place that is a quality about you and not your way in the world. For example, *It's not that I am afraid of rejection; but instead, of course I am afraid of rejection because I believe I am a nobody, and I feel this is so humiliating and shameful.* Notice your body sensations.

2. **Name the ways that you compensate for the core fear.** Try to be honest with yourself about this. It can be difficult.

3. **Externalize the core fear and all the compensations and sensations.** You do this by using your consciousness to peel back all the layers, placing them out in front of you. (Use your imagination to bring them out

in front of you, or make hand motions to lift them out of you—whatever works for you.) If there are any remaining uncomfortable sensations or limiting beliefs (like, *I can't do this*), peel them as well.

4. **Notice that you and the peeled energy are in *Infinite space*.** At infinite acceleration, expand in every direction simultaneously—front, back, above, below, and on both sides of you—and *become the Infinite*. To become the Infinite, most people imagine bursting through the boundary of their skin—moving from being a dense being (in human form) to being expansive like air. Imagine the atoms of your body shooting out so that what was once part of your human body is now part of and dispersed through everything. Many people say that the sensation they feel when they do this can be a feeling like being really high or can be a profound sense of peace. Notice what it is like to be the Infinite. You are likely to feel peaceful, expanded, without boundaries, spacious, and free. If this doesn't happen, if there is any limiting thought, for example, *This will never work for me*, feel the sensation associated with this, peel this off, and expand again until you feel the lightness of being. All of this is who you truly are, your Essence.

5. **Recreate the energy in front of you that was the core fear.** You can do this by simply asking that it return. Ask this energy:

    What is your greatest hope for me?

    What do you wish me to learn in this lifetime (particularly about my purpose)?

    Are there any blessings or anything else you wish to share?

    Will you help me be this hope and learning? (Invariably the answer is yes.)

6. **Notice that in Essence, you already *are* this hope, and that you already know these lessons.** Notice that your greatest fear is, in truth, your greatest good. As you notice this, what happens to the energy that used to be what you called your core fear? Typically, it will totally dissolve again, or

it will turn into something beautiful that will be an anchoring gift for you.

A Case: The Art of Perfection

Rick, a professional artist, told me that he was feeling very agitated and depressed. He had been in a relationship for many years, and his boyfriend had recently broken up with him, citing Rick's criticality and obsessive need to always have everything be "right." Rick was now experiencing extreme self-judgment—even having some suicidal thoughts—although he quickly denied that he would ever consider acting on them. As you may already surmise, Rick was an Enneagram Point 1, the Perfectionist.

The diagnostic revealed that we were to do an Essence Process. I invited Rick to share what he was feeling most ashamed to admit about himself. He told me that he felt ashamed of how critical and righteous he was, and that he believed that he was fundamentally a bad person.

I asked him what he was experiencing in his body as he was allowing that sense of badness. He told me he was feeling sick to his stomach. I invited him to bring all his attention to "sick to stomach," to drop his con-sciousness into it, and to be it. Then, I addressed the sensation directly: "Sick to Stomach, is there anything you are even more afraid to admit about yourself than that you are critical, righteous, and fundamentally bad?"

As Rick started to cry, he reported, "I am so bad that I ought to be in hell, except that there are other people in hell, and I am not even worthy to be with them." With this, he broke down more, saying, "Nothing I ever do will be good enough; I will never get out of this. I hate myself." He seemed to have hit the bottom.

I invited Rick to be aware that while there appeared to be two "I"s, the one who was hating and the one who was hated, there was something else also—the one who was the witness. The hater, the hated, and the badness could not be all of who he was. If they were, he would experience them everywhere in his body, and he could not witness them.

I then suggested to Rick that, while these were perspectives he had about himself, they could not be who he truly was. As Rick understood this, I invited him to take the witness point of view, and, using his consciousness, bring the dense sensation he called "Sick to Stomach" outside of himself so he could observe it.

While he looked at me quizzically at first, he gave me a slight nod, which suggested that he understood me, and then he brought the sensation outside of himself. He said that it was like peeling off a layer that had appeared to be who he was; it now seemed more like a covering. He described it as a dark cloud that he could imagine in front of him.

I invited Rick to notice that the cloud was in a space that was in front of him, behind him, above and below him, to the left and to the right of him. It included him, the cloud, all matter, all energy, and all space. I invited him to expand at an infinite acceleration in all directions, to become the boundaryless, dimensionless, infinitely expanding spaciousness. He was able to do this.

He began to appear radiant and peaceful. He said he was feeling such a sense of serenity. Then, his face took on what, to me, looked like an expression of wonder. Rick said, "I have felt this way once before in my life. It was when I was finishing the one painting with which I felt total satisfaction, my one masterpiece. I doubted that I would ever feel this way again." With this, he started to cry, this time tears of joy.

We asked the energy that used to be his greatest fear what its greatest hope for Rick was. It shared with him that all it ever wanted to do was bring him to the experience of feeling so alive and creating from this place of passion. Rick noticed that he was feeling such aliveness and passion right in that very moment. He looked stunned and grateful that the part of himself that he had so shunned could be his deepest friend and guide.

Several months after this session, Rick reported that it had been life-changing for him to realize that his preoccupation around perfection was preventing him from finding a place of peace and possibility within himself. While he could still feel miserable and neurotic sometimes, and his attention still went to getting things right, he felt more nonattached. He could choose to return to the state of being—which he rediscovered during the session—whenever he thought to, although his feelings may not have been so vivid. He told me that everyone noticed a difference in him, even his former boyfriend. He said that, while it seemed subtle, he truly felt lighter.

Archetypal Identity

As we said earlier, sometimes the compensations for the core fear, the avoidances, take on a life of their own and become highly problematic unto themselves. When this happens, the avoidance is the doorway into finding the core fear, and we call it an Archetypal Identity.

Archetypal Identity occurs when we compulsively live a story that mythologizes our life in order to avoid a deeper fear. We become deeply involved in our relationship to this identity, which comes to take on a life of its own. Any such identity can serve this purpose; it's particularly prevalent with regard to illnesses and addictions. It can also include patterns of relationships and mythical stories. The structure, again, is that an identity masks a fear about ourselves, which masks our True Self. Some examples include:

"I *am* an alcoholic";

"I *am* one who never gets what I want";

"I *am* chronically ill";

"I *am* always a victim";

"I *am* a healer"; and so forth.

Archetypal Identities can be constructive when we let them dance with us and live through us. However, if balancing an Archetypal Identity is indicated, it suggests that the Archetypal Identity has become compulsive and destructive, and is currently serving to avoid a deeper anxiety associated with a core fear.

The key element for healing is that we must ask the identity how it

has developed, how it has served us and limited us, and what is its greatest
fear. For example, an Archetypal Identity of "I *am* a victim" may *serve* us
by allowing us to abdicate responsibility for our life and may also *limit* us
by inhibiting our ability to experiment with new ideas. The key role of the
identity is to cover over a core fear. One possible core fear covered by "I
am a victim" could be that we are dependent and insecure and ultimately
unworthy.

In the case below, the Archetypal Identity is "I am an alcoholic." Notice
how the man discovers how it has both served him and limited him.

A Case: Drinking in Excess for Success

I was working with a high-powered executive named Tom who had
been in alcohol detox several times when he came to see me. We discovered that his statement, "I am an alcoholic," was on one level primarily a
compensation—a story he was telling himself and living out as a way not
to have to experience the anxiety around a fear. I invited him to experience
"I am an alcoholic," and notice what he was feeling in his body. He felt a
deep tightening in his chest. I invited him to bring all his awareness to and
to drop his consciousness into "deep tightening in chest," and to be it and
to let it use his mouth to answer our questions. I asked, "Deep Tightening
in the Chest, how are you trying to serve this being?"

Over the next twenty minutes, it told us the ways it was trying to help
him be a success, both professionally and personally; how it tried to help
him relax, get more done, and be more social; yet it was ashamed because
it was failing. It caused the man to become too relaxed and to sometimes
even fall asleep. He could turn out more work, but the quality of it was
questionable. It became clear that Tom was an Enneagram Point 3, the
Performer, and that the "I am an alcoholic" identity was trying to protect
him from failure while inviting him into it. Our work with this avoidant
identity became the foundation for him to allow his fear of failure.

In this particular case, as he was able to allow this fear, disidentify from it, and then realize his truer self, his drinking released its hold on him for two years. During those two years, he drank nothing. Then, he believed he would be able to enjoy liquor in moderation, and so he started to have a cocktail here and there. He stopped being diligent. This behavior resulted in a relapse. At that point, we redid the Essence work, and he went back to rehab. It seems the combination of the two has kept him clean for fifteen years and running, even to the point where he feels capable of having a drink to celebrate special occasions with no adverse effect. It's important to note here that we are not suggesting that people who have successfully dealt with alcoholism can have an occasional drink. Each case is individual, and people should consult with the professional responsible for their care.

Conclusion

We've done this Essence Process/Archetypal Identity Process with thousands of people, individually and in groups. While not everyone has an experience as immediately and ongoingly powerful as both Rick's and Tom's, most everyone experiences some benefit: a deepening sense of who they are with a lessening attachment to habituated ways of being in the world. This brings a greater sense of choice into everyday life, both around action and meaning making. (Perhaps that Perfectionist can go to sleep one night with the dirty dinner dishes still in the sink and feel fine about it.)

Many of our clients and workshop participants do the Essence Process as an ongoing psychospiritual practice—moving into and disidentifying from deeper and deeper levels of fear. Personally, doing the Essence Process over and over has felt almost like visiting with an old friend and going for a walk with her, each time feeling more love and acceptance for who she is. It has been a path that has loosened the stronghold of our personalities, allowing us to have more freedom of response. It has increased our capacities, each in our own ways, to be more present in Life and to love more purely.

Here's a poem to share that speaks to the process:

Falling Into Grace by A. Hahn

What I want to know is
When you fall,
How do you respond?

Do you pretend you have not fallen?
And if you do,
Do you deny the Grace
That is your place
When you fall?
Do you experience just how small you really are
Or deny the very Essence of the Truth?
And in that act
Deny yourself
And not tend to your garden?

What I want to know is
When you fall,
How do you respond?

Do you frown
Not knowing that you've grown?
Do you groan at the naked pain
And curse the gods as a refrain?
Or do you refrain
From wallowing in the pain,
Experiencing exquisite pain,
A labor
Leading to Creation
Birth?

CHAPTER 13

Opening to All Possibilities for Healing: Times, Dimensions, and Levels

We are almost there. The information that we're sharing can sometimes be a difficult read, and the content can be controversial because it can challenge what we have always known and comfortably relied on as the way life "is." We just have one more topic area to address before we get to the place where you can begin to use this work for yourself, your family, and for therapists, your clients. We hope that you've been intrigued and perhaps even optimistic that what we're sharing, no matter how out of the ordinary it seems, can help you. Now, we're going to turn to a deeper understanding of all times, dimensions, and levels, which will give further insight to the types of stories you may find to facilitate your healing.

To go back to what is fundamental one more time, the key to healing is opening to the intelligence of Life with no presumption about the nature of reality. Therefore, we can make no presumption about the causes of our problem. In that simple lack of presumption, we open to possibilities that we may never have considered both to the nature of our problems and possible resolutions.

Opening to All Times

Most of psychology opens to our problems crystallizing earlier in our current lifetime. While this may be true, there are also other possibilities. As funny as it sounds, although it is rare, sometimes our problems originate either in the future of our current lifetime or in some future beyond our current lifetime. When this is the case, stories we discover feel more like warnings about something that may happen. An analogy might be if we dropped a pebble in the stream of time, we see the ripples/vibration resulting from it go in every direction. From the classical interpretation of time, future traumatic stories feel impossible, but from the perspective of many theoretical physicists who postulate that time is an illusion, future traumatic stories are plausible.

Another possibility is that our stories originate in what is called the time in-between lives. These stories, which are also rare, often have a quality of making some kind of agreement with ourselves and others, but when we get into an actual material life, we find we are unable to keep the covenants for whatever reason. The effect is the same as in everyday life: when we are unable or unwilling to keep these agreements, there are often very traumatic consequences that stem from not living up to or following through with our covenants. What we find is that, as a result of breaking the vow, we either experience quite a setback and have to start all over again, or we have to relearn the lessons that have resulted from the pain others have experienced because of our inability.

More typically, our stories may originate in lifetimes prior to our own. Again, it does not matter if we literally believe in other lifetimes or not. Our only consideration is how useful it is. If we are someone who absolutely cannot open to the possibility of other lifetimes, we then may be able to open to the possibilities of personal mythology, dreams, or imagination.

Myths must reflect the people who created them, and in myths, terribly traumatic things happen. And just as in many cultures that are founded in myth, like Greece, each of us has our own personal mythology.

When we are asleep and we dream, the dream is more real than waking reality in many ways. All the characters in the dream must be, in some way, reflections of ourselves, since we are the creator of the dream. There are often characters in the dream we may never know in waking reality. So, if something very traumatic happens in the dream, on some level, it certainly can reflect something traumatic that we are trying to resolve.

Finally, if nothing else makes sense, we can always open to the imaginal. In child play therapy, children are invited to use their imagination to play out "fictional" scenarios. Another way of understanding what we're doing is the equivalent of play therapy. We are just asking people to focus on the sensation and then use their imagination to let the stories unfold. In our experience, not only do children love telling stories, and we certainly do this with children who come to us for healing, but so do almost all adults.

If we do wish to open to the possibilities of other lifetimes, there is a simple way to do it. From science, we know that once we create energy, even if it fades, it doesn't cease or die. Yet we know that our bodies die. So, what happens to the animating energy that is another name for Soul? Energy that is liberated at our deaths becomes available to be recycled to animate another being. However, that energy is not perfectly "scrubbed clean" and has elements of the experience of the person/persons who utilized it before us.

In the model we are describing, Soul can move through generations in two ways. It can be carried by blood and/or it can be carried by energy. When it is carried by blood, we call the past life *genealogical*. When it is carried by energy, we call the past life *karmic*.

What this means for healing purposes is that if our past life story is genealogical, we are remembering and reliving the lifetime of a particular ancestor or ancestors. If it's karmic, we can be remembering and replaying the story of anything except for our blood ancestors. Occasionally, we are living out both simultaneously, which means that in a karmic past life, we were our ancestor.

In previous chapters, we've already described many sessions that focused on the healing of stories that originated in the karmic past. We will describe two more briefly now because they are so relevant for the whole question of times and dimensions.

In the first case, a man who was a well-known spiritual medium wanted to work on (1) his sense that things didn't turn out right, and (2) some inexplicable and significant stomach problems that were bothering him. It turned out that both equaled a Death Wish, and when he focused on "A part of me wants to die," he felt severe pain in his stomach.

Dropping into "Pain in Stomach," he became aware that he was a train robber in Missouri in the 1870s. During a robbery, he was shot in the stomach and died an excruciatingly slow death. The first thing that was extraordinary to the client was that, even though he knew nothing of this part of American history, he knew exactly what his name was in that lifetime. Researching the name on the Internet, the client discovered there was actually a train robber with this name that died exactly the way he found in the story. He marveled at the fact that, although he communicated with the dead as a medium, it never occurred to him that a dead person in his karmic lineage could be the root cause of his difficulties. He was also able to articulate the difference between the experience of communicating with the dead versus "being" a person who died in another lifetime. He said that communicating with the dead was like inviting a guest in for a talk, while being a person who died in another lifetime was like walking in their shoes and experiencing their life—one that's always been there, but just out of his awareness. He also marveled in a later report that his life seemed qualitatively better and that his stomach problems had abated.

In the second case, many of the client's problems started to resolve when he entered into a lifetime that clearly was his last, where he was a

Nazi general. The client knew very little about Nazism and that period of history. While this general was not particularly well known, there was enough information about him to corroborate all the details that the client found in doing his healing work. And it seemed from where he was now that the general had grown and matured quite a bit in one lifetime.

In a third case, a client found a story about being a soldier in the Pacific Rim during World War II. During the session, he was deeply in the story and at the end calmly looked up and, in a matter-of-fact way, gave the man's name and rank in the Army. At this point, it occurred to the client that the story he found was the same story that he experienced in a recurring dream over a twenty-year period. In the dream, he was running through the jungle, and he would wake in terror not knowing what was happening to him. After accessing the story, where he found he was taken as a prisoner of war and died at the hands of his captors, he never again had the dream.

Several weeks after this session, the client was at the gym with his wife. Remembering the story her husband had told her about the session, she saw a book on the reading table about Guadalcanal in World War II, and she picked it up. There was a list of casualties of war and the person who her husband had named during his session was on the list. She raced over to her husband to show it to him. He stared at the printing on the page in disbelief. Talk about synchronicities!

If a client asks us if they ought to discover if their past life is verifiable by researching information about the story they uncovered, we tell them that it is certainly not necessary for the healing; it's more of a philosophical question. If they feel drawn to discover if what they find is historically verifiable, we invite them to do whatever feels right for them.

We have described far fewer sessions in which the root cause of the problems was genealogical, so we will now turn to a discussion of genealogical past-life stories. Before beginning, we'd like to point out that even though the trauma is carried through the bloodline, it may not literally be carried in a material sense as blood or cellular memory. It can be carried energetically. We believe this because we have encountered cases, such as one in which a grandchild carried a trauma that her grandmother encountered *after* the grandchild's mother was born.

A Spiritual Guide for Our Ancestor's Soul: A Reflection of My Experience with LCT

Until my experience with Life Centered Therapy (LCT), therapy was a performance for me. It was easy because I excelled at saying what I believed others wanted to hear, and if I needed to wear a mask, I could do that, too. Through my work with LCT, I would learn that my body had another story to tell.

I was raised by religious Christian fundamentalists. In this belief system, practitioners adhere to strict—and often oppressive— interpretations of religious thoughts, including ideas regarding the self, others, and the world. My parents were stringent observers of their faith and believed it their duty, ordained by God, to raise us as their disciples.

Part of Christian fundamental ideology encourages disdain for the body, especially the female form. From my mother, I acquired a sense of distrust, hatred, and shame for the body I inhabited. Without a knowledgeable and compassionate guide in my formative years, I never learned how to grow into and explore the dynamic force that I was becoming. By the time I met Joan, I felt detached from my body, the landscape where my heart and spirit ought to dwell. The actions that led me to work with her—people-pleasing, alcohol abuse, and lack of boundaries—affirmed my lack of regard for my body.

In the years since my work with Joan, I often return to a session we had together that radically changed the relationship I had with my body. By then, we had met several times. I had grown accustomed to our initial check-in, followed by muscle testing, which signaled that my performance was over, and the real work could begin. On this particular day, Joan had guided me to a meditative state in which a scene appeared before my closed eyes, but it wasn't like watching a movie. I was a part of it, observing, I believed, unseen.

I saw a small woman, perhaps late twenties to thirties, wearing the clothes of someone from the early twentieth century. She was positioned on her back, nearly lifeless on a sandy, stone floor, save for a look of fear etched across her face. A mustached man glowered above her, poised to strike. He didn't need to, though. There was no blood or noticeable wounds, but it was clear she was on the cusp of death. I sensed it in my own body, an invisible witness to this tragedy unfolding, but also to this woman's life. Suddenly, I felt that the woman knew I was there with her. I perceived her fear like a trembling wave that shot through my body. As her life force faded, I felt another wave, this time, her gratitude for my presence.

I was surprised by the story that came out of my mouth. I had no idea of its origin, except that it began with the tapping of my body (which is an Energy Psychology intervention called Emotional Freedom Technique) . At the time, I knew about historical abuse in both my paternal and maternal lines. However, I had never seen either of the two people in this vision. At the time, when I tried to attach family lore to what I saw, the story became muddled, and my role in it diminished. I decided to let the connection go. Instead, I focused on how this woman felt and how I felt as her witness. By doing so, I was able to discern a feeling in my body I had never felt before. The weight bearing down on my chest had a name: betrayal. Like this woman, I found myself in relationships that drained me of my life force and disempowered me. Also like this woman, I often made myself small to protect myself. In helping her transition, I transformed from the victim I always saw myself as to the psychopomp I was becoming.

The word psychopomp *comes from Greek mythology and refers to someone who is a "guide of the souls," often helping others amid transition. I had long felt a connection to being a Helper, but without healthy boundaries, a clear sense of self, and [having] unresolved trauma, I attracted relationships that sometimes became toxic and/or manipulative and often ended in betrayal.*

You need to have boundaries to be able to work with souls that need guidance. By working with Joan and gaining more awareness of the feelings in my body, I was able to create boundaries. Also, I was finally able to identify the destructive patterns because I relearned how to first sense them in my body. To do this, Joan suggested I focus on cultivating my intuition.

Intuition is stamped out of fundamentalist Christian beliefs because it suggests trusting oneself over its namesake. So, first I had to invite intuition back into my body. Then, I began to incorporate intuitive practices into my life: I embraced tarot, fostered healthy sleeping routines to encourage dreaming, studied and practiced Reiki, meditated, and spent time outdoors. I was also more mindful of the relationships I chose to develop. Naturally, in my waking life, I became more creative, calm, and tuned-in to everything around me. My dreams grew richer in color and story, too.

Five years after my work with Joan, I was back in the US to visit my family. By then, I was happily married and living overseas with my partner. I still culturally identified as Christian but subscribed to a version of the faith that resonated with my values and beliefs. Due to the pandemic, I was unable to return to my home, so I used some of my time to more deeply explore my childhood and my relationship with my mother. I had also connected with a distant cousin, an amateur genealogist, who sent me family photos I had never seen before. When I saw her message with an image of my great-great-grandfather attached, I gasped. It was the man I had seen in my vision with Joan. This was the first photo I had ever seen of him. I quizzed her about him and his wife, who I had learned had disappeared, never to be seen again, when all six of her daughters were under the age of ten. There were no photos of her, just a journalist's description of her around the time of the disappearance that matched the woman in my vision. I decided to tell my cousin about it. The details I shared matched the photos of the family's property, but there was something even more startling. The newspaper article painted her husband in an unflattering, abusive light. Still, the children remained with their father in her absence, and as a result, they grew to resent their mother. She became a woman erased.

My cousin and I pondered the implications of this and wondered what we could do. "We're all in this together. We need our family line to be healed," she told me. At the time, I had decided to transfer my doctoral work in traditional medicine to a North American program. I had been contemplating an area of focus, and I decided to study ancestral healing because, in the end, we are all in this together. I was finally ready to be the psychopomp my great great-grandmother showed me I could be.

—Alys Yves

A Case with Genealogical Root Cause

One of the more powerful genealogical sessions we encountered was not because of the content of the session so much as because of what it revealed about the energetic dynamics of such healings. I was seeing a young man named Seth who was having symptoms of inexplicable fatigue that he believed were somehow related to unexpressed anger. We discovered that the root cause of the issues he was having originated three generations before on his mother's side, and that the fatigue was a protector.

When Seth brought all his attention to fatigue as protector, he had a sensation that he described as a very tight, painful fist in his chest. When he brought all his attention to and became "Tight Painful Fist in Chest," he saw a scene in which a woman was extremely angry at her husband and stuffed it all down. He had a sense that this tightening of the heart eventually showed up as congestive heart failure, which killed her.

He then realized that the reason for his inexplicable fatigue was that he had come back home and had reentered a relationship with his girlfriend. He was stuffing a lot of anger by doing her bidding as opposed to living his own truth. In fact, the fatigue became significantly noticeable when he was asked to mow the lawn and did it. He realized that he had not really made the choice but was just doing it out of a sense of obligation. At the end of the session, his heart felt light and much more energized, and he said that he felt quite certain that if he did something from now on, it would be more because he was choosing to do so as opposed to just going along with things.

When the session was over, as he was walking out to the waiting room to meet his mother who was familiar with LCT, she asked if the session had something to do with her genealogical line. She said that she had noticed a change in her own inner experience during the time that her son was having a session. She had a sense that it had something to do with her grandmother who had died of congestive heart failure. She said that she noticed a lightening in her own heart as he was doing the work. When Seth shared his story with her, she said she hoped that this lightening of heart would allow her to speak up more as well.

It was quite startling to have her reveal her experience. While it doesn't prove anything, it is certainly subjectively suggestive of the transformative power of such genealogical healing work, and that when we are doing our healing work, we potentially are healing not just ourselves, but we can have an impact on the systems and lineages of which we are a part.

Opening to All Dimensions

It's important to understand opening to all dimensions from a practical point of view because it opens us to possibilities for healing that may never have occurred to us. What do we mean by *all dimensions*? Dimensions are simply the different facets of what we perceive to be reality. A simple way to further understand dimensions is the concept of "bandwidths" of vibration. In our work, we discuss seven different *bandwidths*: Elemental, Plant, Animal, Human, Extraterrestrial, Gods and Goddesses, and the Divine (including such beings as guardians, spirit guides, and angels).

In the stories that follow, people who are doing the Life Centered Therapy work identified with beings in each of these bandings. It's important to realize that we can do healings on each of these bandings. As an example, we can do healings on polluted lakes, on sick plants, and on traumatized animals.

Elemental

Sometimes, we discover stories in which we identify with mountains, rocks, or minerals, among other elements. One fascinating example of this occurred at a retreat center. The woman doing the work said that she knew she was going to sound crazy, but that she was both the copper that was strip-mined from the land and the land itself. She told us a story of how she felt she was precious and yet had somehow lost a feeling of home. In her relationships in her current life, she often felt that she was used in a way that almost felt like she was raped and then just left.

From a literal point of view, what was quite extraordinary is that this woman knew nothing about the history of the land of the retreat center, and she told us the next day at the retreat that she had found a book about the history of the center and that there had been copper there that had been strip-mined. From a healing perspective, finding this story was important; when she came to the next retreat, she told us that her relationships were noticeably improved.

Once again, it's important to focus on our *relationship* to these stories. Our bodies help us discover the most powerful and simple stories that lead to our healing and evolution. Whether these stories are literally true or metaphoric is secondary to their healing power. In the case we're describing, it's possible that this woman literally was copper and the land. It is certainly as likely that she was highly intuitively attuned to the copper and the land at the retreat center, and that there was a resonance between what had happened to it and what had happened to her.

Plants

We've had many stories where people have identified with plants, flowers, or trees. Even within the cases in this book, we have heard stories of someone who identified with the healing power of trees and someone who identified as a plant goddess, in this case a wood nymph. We also heard a story in which a tree was cut down in the context of a curse. We've heard many stories of people who have associated with traumatized trees. Sometimes, this includes things like being hit by lightning; other times it includes having limbs cut off with no sense of the impact.

Animals

One particularly compelling session concerned a woman who was constantly feeling the pain of being trapped and an inexplicable shaking sensation.

In her story, she discovered that she was a deer who had gotten caught in a metal trap that snapped shut on her leg. She was shaking from the physical trauma when a hunter came up to her and shot her to death. Healing this story helped her to both physically release the shaking and to psychologically release the theme of being trapped against her will and of being impotent against the power of others.

Human

We obviously have talked at great length about doing healing work with humans and ghosts. So, in this section, we want to focus on a particular kind of human being, ones called empaths.

A Special Case: Empath Healing

While it's still quite unusual, we are finding more people who are coming in for problems that they think are their own but turn out to be the suffering of others. A striking example of this is a woman who came in with unexplainable body discomfort, a sense she was going crazy. A very unusual story that was foundational to all her symptoms originated in a moment when she entered a hospital. We found that she had taken in all the pain that happens in a hospital setting—both the physical and the psychological suffering of the patients, and the sometimes difficult transition from life to death of those who didn't make it.

The key here is that she was not able to distinguish what was hers and what was the pain and suffering of others. When she came to this realization, she was able to do her part to send healing to the people who were suffering, and to help those who needed to transition and go to the Light. Most importantly, which is often the case in empath stories, she needed to strengthen her boundaries so as not to take in what is not hers. After she did this, she reported a noticeable improvement in her suffering because she was more at choice about what she took in.

Extraterrestrials, Gods and Goddesses, Divine Beings

We have talked at some length about beings associated with these bandings earlier in the book in Chapter 9. All that seems important to point out here is that in our sessions, we can identify with human beings who are in relationship with other beings from these dimensions, or we can identify as beings from these dimensions.

Opening to All Energetic Levels

What is the nature of energetic healing? To start with, fundamentally, a symptom means that there is something that couldn't be handled, and, as a result, what was once free-flowing energy (E as in $E = MC^2$) slows down. If energy slows down enough, it becomes matter. We experience the slowed-down energy as a discomfort in our bodies. When we do an LCT session and you/the client chooses to identify with the "witness" who is choosing to *become* the discomfort, you no longer identify with the discomfort; you identify with the one who is with it or hosting it. The traumatic situation that caused the discomfort is no longer something that could not be handled as it is being handled by the host. The discomfort, therefore, returns to its higher vibrational form, which for us means the discomfort dissolves and either all the symptoms or the anxiety associated with the symptoms dissolve.

As we've shown in this book, with awareness, this can be easy to do on your own. So, all we do when we do healing work is align with the energy of Life, the higher vibrational form. In a nutshell, this is all that this book is about. Everything we are teaching you is how to find the most important dense energy to work with (i.e., your stated intention or a pattern), how to find where it originates, and how to find an intervention if aligning with the dense energy is not sufficient to heal.

From the perspective of healing that we just presented, it is useful to think about who we are, not just as a physical body but as energy that comes in three forms: *fields, centers*, and *flows*. We might say that fields are about containers. They are the containers that hold the centers (chakras) and flows (meridians). When the field is integrous, we are whole unto ourselves, and our boundaries are perfectly permeable.

We also have centers of energy. Simply put, centers, whether we talk about them in terms of literal vortices of energy that are called *chakras* (the seven centers of spiritual energy in the human body according to yogic philosophy), or talk about them in terms of modes of perception (head—beliefs; heart—feelings; and belly—boundaries), from our perspective, are about relationships. If we consider *chakras*, they are the bonds that connect us to the communities and larger systems of which we are a part: to creativity, to willingness, to our relationship with others, to our capacity to listen to what is true for us and speak the truth, to our vision, and to all

Life. Further, the relationship between chakras themselves are what create bonds within the field, connecting parts of the fields together.

Finally, we are flows of energy. In Eastern medicine, these flows are called *meridians* (acupuncture works to open our meridians, as does acupressure), and they are like rivers of energy that flow within the fields and between the centers. These rivers are the passageways for information. So, when we are balanced, our fields are whole and coherent, our centers are clear, and we are in the flow.

So why do we come to healers? It follows from our description above that we come for one, two, and/or three reasons. We've had some kind of traumatic shock that has either: (1) fractured the field, leading to the paradox that even though we are here, we feel like we are not all here, or we are disconnected from ourselves; and/or (2) clouded the centers, leading to some kind of relational difficulties; and/or (3) blocked or stagnated the flow, leading to a sense of being frozen, numb, or like the proverbial "deer in the headlights."

Every difficulty that we come to healers to address—be it physical, emotional, mental, relational, or spiritual—is simply one or more of these three energetic variations. From this perspective, it becomes obvious why there is no distinction between mind and body, and that who we are is a mind-body field. Everything that affects the vibration of the mind-body field shows up as symptoms in our body, in our relationship with ourselves, and in our relationship with the world. This explains the truism that our biography is our biology, and our biology is our biography.

The way that we bring our fields back into integrity and coherence, our centers into clarity, and our meridians into flow is to align with the dense energy (matter) as we discussed previously. We might say that this is all healing is, and then everything else is "window dressing" in the service of this. Everything else we do simply makes the healing work more elegant, simple, and powerful.

We presented a lot of ideas in this chapter that may seem foreign to you. In our experience, opening to the possibility that our traumas can originate in any time, dimension, or level can be a useful tool for you on your healing journey. The narrative you learn could be a key to healing the very thing that led you to pick up this book.

We made it through all the material. We've shared all the background information for you to do your own healing work. Let's start!

CHAPTER 14

Using Life Centered Therapy for Your Own Healing

Y ou made it! You can now do the work! You really can! Just breathe and go slowly.

In this chapter, we give you the nuts and bolts of how to do a Life Centered Therapy session on yourself. You can also use the protocol to facilitate LCT for a family member or a friend. While therapists can certainly use the basics of this work with their clients when they feel comfortable, we highly recommend further training to understand the nuances of the work, to work with more difficult populations, and to professionally qualify themselves. (We have a program for people to qualify as a certified practitioner.)

> Disclaimer: The Life Centered Therapy protocol provided in this book should not be used by or for anyone who has these symptoms: delusions, hallucinations, periods of time in your life that you can't account for, and suicidal ideation. Also, if you have a diagnosis of substance abuse disorders, dissociative identity disorder (DID), borderline personality disorder (BPD) with any psychotic features, schizophrenia and or other psychotic disorders, you should *not* use this protocol. To use the protocol in this book, these symptoms and diagnoses require the support of a mental health professional who is an LCT certified practitioner and are beyond the scope of this self-help book.

Before beginning a healing, it's a good idea to do a *centering practice*. You can do this by bringing your awareness down and into the body, and following your breathing for several breaths. Set the intention to open your Head Center to true wisdom and vision, your Belly Center to knowing what is true for you and what is most important to share, and your Heart Center to the soft voice that knows what you truly desire. Then, it's almost as if you are sharing answers from a deeper part of you. Stay in this space and speak slowly enough that you are literally *listening* to what this deeper part of you is sharing with you. Stay focused in the body throughout your entire session.

There are two ways that you can do your own healing. The first is the simplest.

First Method of LCT Healing

Find something that you are suffering about. Let yourself fully experience the suffering, scan your body, and notice the sensations that arise. Choose to bring all your attention to the sensations so that you *become* the sensation from the inside out. Ask the sensation, "What have you come to share? Where are you beginning? What is happening?" Be receptive. (Some people find it useful to write down their story or record it.) When you sense that you have the whole story, if some discomfort still remains, it's likely that you need an *intervention*. Find an intervention, either intuitively or by looking at the list in this chapter along with how to do each one). If using the list, you can muscle test if you're comfortable doing that. While focusing on the discomfort, do the intervention until complete (you'll know it's complete when your discomfort is gone, and you feel a sense of peace). This completes the process. Reflect on what you discovered and what you learned. Check in with yourself and see each day if you notice a difference in what you worked on.

Feet flat on the floor. Letting the breath flow through me. Bringing the gaze in and down. Scanning the body. Connecting with the open heart, the knowing belly, and the clear-sighted mind.

What is asking for my attention? If I could receive anything in the world right now, what would it be? What am I here to share?

I came to this practice because I was stuck and miserable, and I couldn't name why. I was in pain on multiple levels. Traumas I had tucked away, anxieties so constant that they'd become my default, and the hunger to be fully present all clamored for my attention once I started doing this work. However, the incredible beauty of LCT is the way that being with your pain becomes your path home. It takes what is already there (a repressed memory or a self-negating belief) and shakes it out so you can see it. The work is your safety net. Whatever comes through is only there because you are ready to take care of it.

Over the ten months that I dove deep with LCT, I experienced searing pain and indescribable grace during each visit. Sometimes, years of misalignment snapped instantly into place once I allowed my pain to share its story. Sometimes, I revisited a memory from multiple angles, over many tear-filled sessions, before sensing a bigger shift. Sometimes, nothing seemed to happen at all, until the exact situation I most needed for healing appeared in my life a few days later. Life Centered Therapy taught me to trust in the magic within and around me and to embody that magic in the moments between the sessions.

The more faith I held in myself for answers, the more my brightness flowed outward toward other people in my life, illuminating their own starlight and shadow. Life Centered Therapy is an ongoing journey of love. If you have found it, welcome. I wish you the courage to see yourself as a constellation, too: blazingly bright and inky black all at once. The darkness within you is nothing to fear; as this practice teaches, it's only in accepting all of who we are and in embracing the contrasts therein that our light can be seen.

—Kelly R.

The second way to do your own self-healing is to follow the protocol that is provided further in this chapter.

Through a specific template protocol that includes attunement and a combination of kinesiology and intuition, the source of the issue is discovered to work with. Then, I go to a deep place within myself and sense or see the origin story. For me, this was sometimes sensed somatically (i.e., in the body) and at other times visually (like watching a movie in my mind's eye). For some issues, the source issue proved to have occurred during this lifetime, and for a number of issues, the origin was from other lifetimes of my soul. A number of those involved energetically and emotionally completing past deaths that were not only believable to me, but that I truly embodied and sensed as each one cleared. The healing modalities included in this therapy are an encyclopedic resource of energy healing modalities that could be done with simple instruction. The process of multiple healings can be compared to gently removing layers of an onion that no longer serve or belong attached to our souls.

This therapy taught me skills and awareness including: (1) the ability to sense, through the body, how an emotion or thought was manifesting and then, through quiet acceptance, to allow it to pass with awareness; (2) a realization that what is manifesting in our lives in the present is connected to all time for our soul and on levels broad as well as deep; (3) that time is truly an illusion; (4) to have the awareness and ability to access aspects of ourselves heretofore inaccessible by both a lack of awareness and of skill; and finally, (5) the process gave me the priceless gift of compassion for myself and others.

—Debra L. Glasser, MD,
Internal Medicine

Gems

As we prepare to do a session, here are a few "gems" that we invite you to remember to help you get through the process.

1. Everything is part of the process.

Once you begin a "session," everything becomes part of the process. From the moment you start, be curious about everything that you say, everything that you notice, and everything that happens to you. This is true even about statements or beliefs that you might be sure are content reflections about your process in the here and now.

One of Joni's ongoing clients came in for a session after having major surgery. She said she was so much looking forward to the session because she had many concerns about her health and was experiencing a sense of depression. When I asked her what she would like from our time together, she had difficulty answering because she said, though she was embarrassed to admit it, she was feeling distracted by a conversation that she had had earlier in the day with a friend about the new shade of red that she had dyed her hair. She was wondering if her hair was the "right" color. As the session unfolded, it turned out that we were to work on the anxiety she experienced as she ruminated about whether the hair color was the right one. Through exploring this anxiety, we learned that what she really was concerned about was whether, after a surgery that left her partially disabled, she would ever be able to feel playful again. She saw the new hair color as an expression of her playfulness, and, therefore, felt it might no longer be appropriate. So, the "distraction" was really the doorway into the very deep work that was essential for her in that moment.

This realization becomes even more salient in the third step of the process in which we "find the story." We often make statements that convey beliefs that we are sure are statements about the here and now. To give an obvious example, suppose you are working and say, "I can't do this." Invariably, we will discover a story where you can't do something. In a similar vein, suppose you say, "I can't see anything." What you may believe you mean is that you are unable to do this process because no images are coming to you. It is much more likely that you are in a story where you can't see anything. If this, in fact, is the case, you can gain movement by reminding yourself that you're in a memory, and in that memory, you can't see anything. We continually encounter examples of this, and it's the realization that these content-level statements are a part of the narrative itself that each time powerfully moves the process forward. This is a crucial point in the decision-making of the flow of any session. If we move to exploring the "problem," or to the metaphoric, or to self-doubt, and miss the opening, the session will invariably go off track. Staying in the concrete and literal will invariably bring us home.

So, if a person you are working with (or even if you're doing the work with yourself) does say something like, "I can't see anything," technically a correct response is, "Yes, you can't see anything, and…" Or, alternatively, if you are exactly mirroring, then you can say, "Yes, I can't see anything, and…"

2. Listen in the literal.

It's profoundly important to listen literally to what you or the client says as opposed to listening metaphorically. If someone describes their depression as making them feel weighed down, helpless, and hopeless like Sylvia in Chapter 5, it's not a metaphorical way of describing her depression. It's a literal narrative that she is revealing through her very wording. If someone says in a session, "I fell into something," it is likely they are in a story where they literally fell into something—like a well. The literal language again is profoundly important. It's fundamental to respond to the literal language only and not to paraphrase or presume meaning.

> *I was experiencing an intense dizziness and headache. It was interfering with my work and a deadline at the end of the week–I had just three days left to get the editing work done that I had*

promised Andy and Joni. The task was overwhelming before the dizziness and headache, but with those physical symptoms slowing me down, my stress level increased.

I called Andy, and he asked me to identify the physical sensations. I said it was a terrible dizziness or vertigo, and that I felt pressure in my temples as well. I then asked, "Pressure in temples and dizziness, what have you come to share? Where are you beginning? What's happening?" I sat with my eyes closed, but I saw nothing, heard nothing, felt nothing. My panic increased. I felt like I was wasting valuable time that I should be spending working. I said, "I don't want to waste time; I should just go. There's not enough time." And Andy said, "Yes, that's right–you're on the right track. Keep going."

This perplexed me. I thought I should get off the phone, and he wanted me to keep talking about how this was wasting time! But I played along and tried to quiet my mind. Still seeing nothing in my mind's eye, my frustration increased. "I really need to get back to work and work faster. This material is so dense, and I'm worried I won't get through it all in time. There's not enough time. I'm just not working fast enough. I'm so overwhelmed—it's dizzying." I was thinking Andy would pick up on the cue that I needed to get off the phone then, but he just calmly said, "That's right—there's not enough time. What is happening next?"

I shook my head and thought, nothing is happening next. I'm in my office. But then, I saw the word "college" appear on the screen in my mind. This was so confusing to me. I said, "College—something about college." And Andy said, "Yes, that's right." So, I suddenly said, "I can't wrap my mind around the material—it's so dense. There's so much pressure, and the clock is ticking. I'm so worried about failing."

Long story short—my dizziness and headache were my body's physical representation of my stress. I'm apparently very literal in my stress. I even said that my overwhelm was "dizzying." I also said, "There's so much pressure." That became pressure in my head—a headache. I also said that I was struggling to "wrap my head around" the material. Funny enough, the headache radiated from my temples around my head. I don't know what specific event in college I was remembering, but I do remember the feeling. That was all I needed to alleviate the vertigo/dizziness and headache and get back to work.

—Meghan Hill

3. The body never lies.

Focus on your body experience; you will always get where you need to go when you do this. In our experience, as soon as you try to "figure something out," you can be easily led astray. Sometimes, the body sensations you need to find are immediately accessible to you. At other times, you might need help finding them by making some statement (restating your blocked intention and/or the core experience of one of the patterns) that will help you find the sensation(s). Whether we start with the body sensation or the statement which helps us find it, our ultimate intention is to be actively receptive to the sensation(s) and to the story and experiences they hold. Once you focus on the wisdom of the body, you become the expert reporter of the sensation's experience, whoever that is. In this way, you often know exactly what you need to heal. This realization can be very empowering for people.

4) Matrices of beliefs shift simultaneously.

Often, we believe that we have to work on one problem at a time. From a much broader perspective, we discover that problems that are seemingly unrelated may all be enfolded into some organizing narrative.

Again, remember the story of Sylvia in Chapter 5. Who would have guessed that her chronic neck pain, which she hadn't even thought to mention, her fear of being in front of crowds, her helplessness, her depression, and even her inability to feel God's presence were surface structures that were enfolded into one archetypal narrative? And who would have guessed that by transforming that story of an unfinished death, a couple of minutes later she would be standing in front of the whole crowd with no anxiety, a sense of lightness that she hadn't remembered ever feeling, an ability to easily move her neck without pain, and a felt sense of the Divine?

The significant point here is that the details of the narrative can be important in terms of your life and the symptoms that you live with, even if those symptoms were not in your conscious awareness when beginning the session.

5. Always ask first if you or your Partner 'knows' what they need.

In our experience, more often than not, the person doing the work *does* know. And, if they didn't know that they knew, then realizing that they did is a great gift. Moreover, if it turns out that they in fact did not know, this, too, can be extremely liberating because they no longer have to blame themselves for not being able to resolve the difficulty. We do this as a way of honoring the deep self-wisdom within each of us. Further, by accessing this wisdom, people become more aware of it and begin to trust themselves more.

Overview of the Five-Step Process

Before beginning, it's helpful to understand the five-step process. Simply put, you will:

1. Find the most important intention to work on and determine if it is safe to work on it.

2. Determine if you need to include one of the patterns as part of your work.

3. Find out if you need information about the story, and, if you do, find it. And find out if you need an intervention and, if you do, find it.

4. After experiencing the block on your intention, drop into the body sensation that arises and find the story. Do the intervention, if called for.

5. Discover lessons and ongoing practices to get the full benefit from the work.

The protocol is a decision tree of primarily yes and no answers. It leads you to where you need to go and is quite easy to follow as long as you stay focused. We first explain each step. Then, we provide the list of questions for each step after the brief explanations.

Step One: Finding the Highest Priority Intention, and Safety Checks

In this step, you find the Highest Priority Intention (HPI). This means discovering what is the most important issue(s) to address that will maximize the benefit of the work (think of healing work as peeling an onion, layer by layer). The person who is doing the work creates a list of issues they would like to work on. This list can include, for example, things like wanting to lose ten pounds, wanting to be able to complete writing a book they have been working on for some time, or wanting to fully forgive a parent for something that happened in childhood.

The list is different for everyone, and the possibilities are endless. You then muscle test to discover if the client knows their HPI, and if they don't, you muscle test the list to find out what is the most important issue(s) to address. After determining the HPI, you must determine if it is safe to do the work and if all parts of you, if you are working alone, or of the person doing the work whom you are facilitating, give permission to proceed.

The protocol that follows provides the questions to muscle test to make this determination. Step One is complete when the HPI is determined, the safety checks are completed, and all parts give permission to do the work.

Step Two: Check for Patterns

In this step, you find out whether to work only on the stated intention you found in Step One or if you also need to work with a theme of a pattern in order to get the best result. (Remember John in Chapter 6 with the bombs going off in the Afghan war. His real problem is the betrayal of trust, and he needed that information to get to the real problem.) Step Two is complete when you have determined if working with a pattern(s) is necessary, and if so, you have identified the relevant pattern(s).

Step Three: How to Find the Story and the Intervention

In this step, you discover if you need to find out information about the root cause story that underlies the trauma. Sometimes, all you need to do is to drop into the body sensation associated with the HPI and let it reveal its story, and no other information is needed. Other times, you need to discover information about the story before dropping in. Did it occur in this lifetime? What age? Another lifetime? Who or what are you in the story? Where did it take place? (Remember the woman who had an accident at the ocean in Chapter 2, and the root cause was a story about being a Roman general 2,000 years earlier. For Nate, who was depressed in Chapter 5, the root cause was before five years old in this lifetime.)

After discovering information about the story, you then determine if, additionally, a practice or intervention is needed in order to balance the intention, that is, get unstuck. We have included nine common interventions taken from the world of energy psychology. However, one of the reasons Life Centered Therapy is so powerful is because, by its design, it's set up to incorporate the best of all other frameworks. It does not prescribe practices/interventions. If an intervention is called for, you are invited to open to an essentially unlimited number of intervention possibilities and choose the one that will most effectively release the block. You might find the intervention intuitively or use something from another healing approach. Step Three is complete when you've found the information you need to access the story, and if an intervention(s) is called for, you have identified the intervention(s) to release the block and get unstuck.

Step Four: Balancing the Block on the Intention—Finding the Story and Doing the Intervention

In this step, the actual healing work occurs. To find the story that is blocking the intention, you need to find the body sensation associated with this blocked intention. The way to do this is to bring all of one's attention to the block in the HPI. If the HPI is stated as a block, a negative (e.g., "I want to remove the block from writing my book"), then you are invited to drop into the sensation associated with "Something is blocking me from writing the book." If the intention is worded in the positive ("I want to finish writing my book"), then you want to feel in the body *how* you are unable to finish writing the book. The idea here is to activate that which is blocking you from manifesting what you want in the world.

In the case where you find a pattern in Step Two that's important to finding the story, you also want to allow yourself to experience the core theme of the pattern along with the block on the stated intention. As an example, if the intention is wanting to finish writing my book and a Violence Pattern was identified in Step Two, I would want to bring all of my attention to not being able to finish writing the book *and* to feeling vulnerable in the world. After opening to these two experiences, I then want to notice what is happening in the body.

After finding the sensation, bring all your attention to the sensation and let it share its story. Whatever the sensation shares *is* the story. Be aware that the story may reveal itself through auditory, visual, or kines-thetic channels. When in auditory mode, you will hear the story; in visual mode, you will see the story; and in kinesthetic mode, you may only feel more body sensations, for example, "I am falling back," or perhaps, "My arms are getting tired." As long as the attention stays on the sensation(s), trust that what is revealing itself is the right thing.

When the sensation(s) have fully shared, and if a practice or inter-vention is called for, do the intervention. Step Four is complete when the full story has been found, the intervention is done, and the block on the intention is balanced. The way you will know for sure that something is balanced is that you will sense this in your body. The sensation that was associated with the blocked intention will dissipate. You are likely to also have a subjective experience of things "being in right order."

Step Five: Conclusion: Integrating the Healing into Your Life

In this step, you are invited *into* what you have learned from the heal-ing. In addition, any pragmatic changes that would support the healing are identified. These may include any habits to be released, behavioral changes to identify, any ongoing affirmations that may be useful, and so forth. The key is to find whatever is necessary to create a positive and lasting impact in your life. You are then asked to affirm the healing, meaning that you accept a new way of being in your life with all the changes, responsibilities, and accountability that accompany that shift. Step Five is complete when you have accessed all the learnings, identified all changes that need to happen to support the new way of being in the world, and affirmed the balance.

The Simple Five-Step Healing Protocol

You'll need paper and a pen/pencil when you do this work. Sometimes people like to keep a notebook of their sessions so they can refer to earlier sessions or review their progress.

Before beginning to do the work for yourself or with a partner we suggest that you bring yourself fully into the moment. A way to do this is to bring awareness down and into the body and follow your breathing for several breaths. Set the intention to open your Head Center to true wisdom and vision, your Belly Center to knowing what is true for you and what is most important to share, and your Heart Center to the soft voice that knows what you truly desire. Then, it's almost as if you're sharing answers from a deeper part of you. Stay in and speak slowly enough that it is like you are literally listening to what this deeper part of you is sharing. Stay focused in the body throughout your entire session.

In the protocol below:

- MT indicates a prompt to muscle test. (Remember muscle testing is binary; it gives yes/no answers.)

- **Bold, *italicized*** words are questions you ask or statements you make to yourself or your healing partner.

- When you MT a question, it will most often be followed by "If yes" and "If no," which gets you further into the decision tree. This is indicated by the indents in the formatting.

STEP I: FINDING THE HIGHEST PRIORITY INTENTION (HPI) AND SAFETY CHECKS

1.0. Before beginning the body of the protocol, it's important to check muscle testing for yes/no answers. You can do this by asking the body to:

> MT • ***Give me a yes.*** This answer is the body's yes. Typically, the muscle stays strong.

> MT • ***Give me a no.*** This answer is the body's no. Typically, the muscle weakens.

If the muscle weakens with a yes, then it ought to stay strong for a no.

Once you have established the body's yes/no answers, you can proceed to Question 1.1.

Things to remember when muscle testing:

- Set the intention to connect with the deepest level of knowing, and ensure that the information you receive is in the service of your/ your healing partner's highest good and Soul evolution.
- Relinquish attachment to outcome.
- Stay open and curious.
- Slow down and notice your energy; keep it down and in.
- Muscle test with the same firmness every time.
- Push until you feel the muscle lock.
- Pause after asking a question so the body has time to react.
- Be attentive to muscle fatigue and hydration.
- If muscle testing another, MT dominant arm if there is nothing to contraindicate this (like a shoulder problem). When fatigued, you can switch arms
- Avoid using the word "should" as it suggests right/wrong; use "is" or "ought" instead, as neither suggest judgment.

FINDING THE HIGHEST PRIORITY INTENTION

1.1. *If you could have anything you desire from our time together, even if it seems like a miracle, what would you intend?*

Number and write down each intention exactly as stated whether you are working alone or with a partner.

1.2. MT • *Is the Highest Priority Intention (HPI) any, some, and/or all of the intentions on the list?*

You are likely to work on just one intention. Or, occasionally, several intentions on the list may be all part of one HPI. You will MT to determine how many of the intentions are the HPI, MT to see if the client knows the HPI and if no, then MT to discover which one(s) to work with.

If no, MT • *Is the HPI one of the patterns?*

> **If yes,** MT the list of patterns to find out which is the HPI.
>
> You do this by first MTing if it is a Single-Center Pattern, Triple-Center Pattern, or an Identity Pattern. The list of patterns and their inducting statements appears at the end of Step I.
>
> MT until you get a yes: *Is a Single-Center Pattern the HPI? Is a Triple-Center Pattern the HPI? Is an Identity Pattern the HPI?* Once you know the category of pattern, then determine which pattern in the category it is by **MT** • *Is [name pattern] the HPI?* and so forth. Continue until you get a yes answer. Then, proceed to question 1.3.

We have given you the inducting statements for all the patterns, and you can use those inducting statements as the highest priority intention. We have included enough information in the overview of each of the patterns (we suggest you read the one specific to the healing you are doing) to enable you to facilitate the healing. While there are other technical considerations that we teach in our trainings about each pattern, there is sufficient information included in the pattern explanation in this book to support you in getting excellent results. We include a link to our website, www.LifeCenteredTherapy.com, to find resources that are available to support you in your ongoing learning.

> **If no,** either find the HPI intuitively, or find out what resource to use to find it. (Resources might include books, for example, *You Can Heal Your Life* by Louise Hay, or it might be a person you know, or lyrics from a song.) If you are working with a partner, **MT** • *Do they find it? Do you find it? Do you talk about it?*

If yes, MT • *Do I* (if working alone) *or does the client know the HPI?*

> **If yes,** if working alone, just go inside and find out which you are to work with. If working with another person, tell them they know what their HPI is, and they can go inside and find it.

If no, MT • *Is the HPI just one of the intentions on the list?*

If yes, MT the list to find out which is the HPI.

You do this by asking:

> MT • *Is intention one the HPI?* Followed by **MT–*Is intention two the HPI?*** Continue until you get a yes answer. Then proceed to Question 1.3.

If no, then the HPI is more than one of the intentions on the list.

MT • Is the HPI all of the intentions on the list?

> **If yes,** the HPI is everything that was said.

> **If no,** MT • *Is the HPI two of the intentions on the list?* Followed by **MT–*Is the HPI three intentions on the list?*** Continue until you get a yes answer.

Once you know the number of intentions that comprise the HPI, you then need to MT the list to determine which ones they are. For example, if there are six intentions on the list, and two of them are the HPI, you MT each intention, starting with the first until you get a yes to two intentions.

> MT • *Is intention one part of the HPI? Is intention two part of the HPI?* You continue this questioning until you get yes to the number of intentions that comprise the HPI.

1.3. MT • *Is the intention worded exactly correctly?*

If yes, proceed to Question 1.4.

If no, find the right wording, and MT new wording by asking Question 1.3 again. Keep refining wording until the answer to Question 1.3 is a yes.

It's important to determine if the HPI is worded exactly correctly. Sometimes, you need to add information or take information away. As an example, if the stated HPI is "I want to not be angry with my mother," and this HPI is not worded correctly, it may be because you are invited to work on your anger in general and not just with your mother. The correct wording might be, "I want to not be angry in the world."

1.4. MT • *Are we to identify how you will know the balance has worked?*

If no, proceed to Question 1.5.

If yes, this is called ensuring the intention is quantifiable. Ask: *How will your life be different once your intention is balanced?* Write down your answer.

As an example, if the HPI is, "I want a happier life," it's important to determine what a happier life would look like and how you would know when you achieved it.

SAFETY CHECKS: PERMISSION TO DO THE WORK

1.5. MT • *Do all parts give 100 percent permission to do this balance?*

- Generally, the answer is yes.
- If the answer is no, you need to find the part that does not give permission.
  - Speaking directly to that part, invite it to share. Sometimes, all the part needs is to express its concern about proceeding.

If yes, proceed to Question 1.6.

If no, invite the part that does not give permission to proceed to share its concern, and then ask:

> **MT •** *Do all parts now give 100 percent permission to do this balance?*
>
> > **If yes,** proceed to Question 1.6
> >
> > **If no,** MT • *Shall we do a balance on the part that does not give permission?*
> >
> > > **If yes,** this becomes your new HPI–doing a balance on the part that doesn't give permission.
> > >
> > > **If no,** MT • *Is there anything we are to do so that this part gives permission?*
> > >
> > > > **If yes,** discover what to do and do it.

If no, STOP WORK FOR THE DAY. All parts need to give permission to proceed with the work.

1.6. MT • *Any reason not to proceed?*

If no, the safety checks are now complete, and you can proceed to Step II, Question 2.1.

If yes, determine the reason not to proceed (see below) by checking in with yourself or your partner, and then take corrective action that allows you to proceed. Then ask Question 1.6 again. The answer ought to be no.

Asking if all parts give permission is asking deepest wisdom to give permission to do the work. Any reason not to proceed may be something simple like having to take a moment to sit with your fear before continuing, taking a bathroom break, or even just having a snack before starting.

PATTERNS AND THEIR CORE EXPERIENCES	
SINGLE CENTER PATTERNS	CORE EXPERIENCE–INDUCTING STATEMENT
Head	The reverse/conflicted belief is the inducting statement
Heart	I am afraid to experience/express (fill in feeling)
Belly	I am not at choice around my boundaries about (fill in boundary)
TRIPLE CENTER PATTERNS	CORE EXPERIENCE–INDUCTING STATEMENT
MATERIAL REALMS	
Split/Multiple	A part of me is missing/I'm not all here/I don't have all my energy/ Part of me feels disconnected from another part of me/I feel fragmented.

TRIPLE CENTER PATTERNS	CORE EXPERIENCE–INDUCTING STATEMENT
Power	I spoke/acted my truth and I was oppressed/ostracized/silenced because of it.
Death Wish	A part of me wants to die/A part of me wishes I was dead/Someone who is supposed to love me wants me dead; in order to receive their love, a part of me has to die.
Fractured Boundaries	Nothing sticks inside/Nothing nourishes me/I leak out of myself/ I am an empty husk/ No one is at home.
Grudge	My values have been violated, and I act in a way that will guarantee they will continue to be violated.
Neglect	When I really needed you as if my life depended on it, you were not there for me.
Wounded	I have betrayed.
Double Bind	If I get what I want, something even worse will happen than if I don't get what I want, and my reality about this will be denied.
Major Loss Trauma	I feel empty.
Major Violence Trauma	I feel vulnerable/I feel polluted.
Already Dead Parts	Part(s) of me is/feels numb or already dead.
Blocked	I'm afraid if I experience (remember), I will be overwhelmed/shattered.
Individuation Trauma	I feel separate from Source.

TRIPLE CENTER PATTERNS	CORE EXPERIENCE–INDUCING STATEMENT
Fear of Loss of Self in Relationship	I am unable to handle the anxiety that accompanies being in a relationship with you. Therefore, I defuse the anxiety by sabotaging by (choose all that apply) compulsively making myself too distant, making myself too close, going on automatic in the relationship, or bringing in some-thing else (person or thing).
Seduction • Seducer • Seducee	To feel alive, I seduce others. To feel alive, I let others seduce me.
Wonderful	I long for what I've had. I compulsively seek to recreate it, destroying what I have.
NONMATERIAL REALMS	
Entity	Something is attached to me and draining my energy.
Ghost	Someone is attached to me and draining my energy.
Curse	I am or feel cursed. Or, I am cursing.
Superimposition	Something much bigger than me is holding me back, keeping me down, or has taken me over.
Extraterrestrial • Implant • Abduction • Walk-in • Identified with extraterrestrial	I feel I am being experimented on; controlled by outside forces. I have been taken against my will. Some energy has pushed me aside and taken over my body. I am an extraterrestrial and something is wrong.

IDENTITY PATTERNS	CORE EXPERIENCE–INDUCING STATEMENT
Blocked Identity	The protecting, obscuring limiting identity typically found in the check-in[1]
Embodiment Identity	Statement of the core fear
Archetypal Identity	The way we compensate for the core fear.

STEP II: CHECKING FOR PATTERNS

In Step II, if the highest priority intention in Step I is not a pattern but something that was said, you need to check if you need to work with a pattern as well as the stated intention. If the highest priority intention was a pattern, you can skip this step.

2.1 MT • *Are we to work with a pattern?*

> **If no,** proceed to Step 3, Question 3.1.
>
> **If yes,** MT the list of patterns to find out which you are to work with in addition to working with the HPI. You will put the two together to form one intention. The list of patterns and their inducing statements appear just before Step II.
>
> > You do this by first MT if it is a Single-Center Pattern, Triple-Center Pattern, or an Identity Pattern.
> >
> > > MT until you get a yes: *Is a Single-Center Pattern the HPI? Is a Triple-Center Pattern the HPI? Is an Identity Pattern the HPI?* Once you know the category of pattern then determine which pattern in the category it is by **MT–*Is (name pattern) the HPI?*** Continue until you get a yes answer. Then, proceed to Question 3.1.

---

[1] In the case of Nate, "I'm depressed/I don't care" that was found in the check-in.

We have given you the inducting statements for all of the patterns and you can use those inducting statements along with the highest priority intention found in Step I. We have included enough information in the overview of each of the patterns (which we suggest you read the one specific to the healing you are doing) to enable you to facilitate the healing. While there are other technical considerations that we teach in our trainings about each pattern, there is sufficient information included in the pattern explanation in this book to support you in getting excellent results. We include a link to our website, www.LifeCenteredTherapy.com to find resources that are available to support you in your ongoing learning.

STEP III: FINDING INFORMATION ABOUT THE STORY AND IDENTIFYING THE INTERVENTION

FINDING OUT ABOUT THE STORY

3.1. MT • *Are we to find out anything about the story (narrative) through MT?*

> **If no,** proceed to Question 3.2.
>
> **If yes,** MT • *Do we find out what lifetime?*
>
>> **If yes,** MT • *Present life? Past life? Future life?*
>>
>>> **If present life,** MT • *Do we find out what age?*
>>>
>>>> **If yes,** MT age.
>>>
>>> **If past or future,** MT • *Karmic? Genealogical?*
>>>
>>>> • Karmic stories are stories that come through an energetic line, while genealogical stories pass down through the bloodline.
>>>>
>>>> • If you or the person you are working with is uncomfortable with the idea of past lives or future lives, think of them as imaginal stories—undreamed dreams.

3.2. MT • *Anything else to find out about the story through muscle testing before proceeding?*

If no, proceed to Question 3.3.

If yes, MT • *Do we have to find when? Where? People involved? Etc.* When you have to find this additional information, you or the person you are working with is invited to go inside and find the possibilities of answers to the questions. MT these possibilities. Keep finding information and re-asking Question 3.2 until the answer is no.

IDENTIFYING THE INTERVENTION

Part of the power of Life Centered Therapy is that it's an inclusive framework that doesn't prescribe what you need to do but invites you to open to all of Life, including other practices from other approaches, or ones of your own making, to shift energy and heal. We often know intuitively what we need to resolve our difficulties. The first place for us to look for practices or interventions within ourselves: just tune into our hearts, be receptive, and see what comes to us. In our experience, people we work with frequently know what they need. If they don't know what they need, we provide a list of nine commonly used interventions. Question 3.4 below asks if you are to find the intervention intuitively or to use one of the interventions provided below.

3.3 MT • *Do we need to find an intervention?*

If no, proceed to Question 4.1.

If yes, find the intervention. MT • *Is it one intervention made up of one?*

If yes, proceed to Question 3.4.

If no, MT • *Is it one made up of more than one?*

If yes, MT • *Is it made up of two and only two? Three and only three?* Stop when you get a yes answer. An intervention made up of more than one intervention is usually two interventions that you do at the same time. An example of this may be to do an intervention called frontal occipital holding (FOH) while channeling Light (one intervention made up of two: FOH and Light).

After identifying the number of interventions that make up the one intervention, proceed to Question 3.4.

If no, MT • *Is it more than one?* (The answer to this ought to be yes.)

>**If yes,** MT • *Is it two and only two? Is it three and only three?* Stop when you get a yes answer. After identifying the number of interventions, proceed to Question 3.4. If the intervention is more than one, you usually identify several interventions and do them sequentially. You might do FOH, and when that is complete, do Light.

3.4. MT • *Do we access the intervention(s) by muscle testing the list?*

If yes, MT the list, making sure you are aware of how many interventions you need to identify. Start at the top of the list and **MT** • *Is intervention one part of the intervention? Is intervention two part of the intervention?* You continue this questioning until you get yes to the number of interventions that comprise the overall intervention, or the number of interventions you need to do.

If no, MT • *Do I access it/them intuitively?* The answer to this ought to be yes.

>**If yes,** access it/them intuitively by either looking within and sharing whatever comes to you, even if it makes no conscious sense, or by looking at the list and not muscle testing it but choosing what feels right.

>**If no,** you need to get creative. You need to find what resource it is in.

LIST OF INTERVENTIONS (INSTRUCTIONS FOLLOW LATER IN CHAPTER.)

Frontal Occipital Holding (FOH)

Stress Release

Fear Points

Anger Points

Shame Points

Boundary Tapping

Reversal Tapping

Letting Go

Light

STEP IV: FINDING THE STORY AND DOING THE INTERVENTION

4.1. If the intention includes a pattern, (1) and it is only a pattern, say the inducting statement of the pattern out loud (2) if the intention includes a stated intention *and* a pattern, say the stated intention and inducting statement of the pattern out loud.

Feel the uncomfortable sensations associated with the blocked intention.

> If the stated intention is framed in the positive, you want to focus on what *not* achieving that feels like in the body. If the intention names the block, you want to focus on what that feels like in the body. We want you to feel what is blocking you.
>
> > Example: Intention–Be a powerful public speaker
> >
> > Focus on sensations associated with "Something is blocking me from being a powerful public speaker."
> >
> > Example: Intention–Balance depression
> >
> > Focus on sensations associated with depression.

4.2. Write down whatever body sensations you are experiencing. Include where you are experiencing them in the body. Examples include weak knees, nausea, heavy or racing heart, tears, etc. If you feel nothing, you are experiencing a feeling of "feeling nothing." If you are feeling nothing, fully allow, "I am feeling nothing," and notice where in the body you are feeling, "I am feeling nothing."

4.3. Drop awareness into these sensations, meaning bring all your focus to them as if you are the sensations. Speaking directly to the sensations by naming them, ask them what they have come to share. You may ask the sensation(s): *Who/what are you? Where are you beginning? What is happening? and/or What have you come to share?*

- Be available through all senses. You might become the being who is having the sensation (kinesthetic), imagine the story in your mind's eye (visual), and/or hear words/have ideas (auditory). Just report whatever you are experiencing, feeling, imagining, sensing, and thinking.

- Assume that everything that comes up is part of the story, and not just a statement of your current experience. For example, if you are experiencing something like, "I can't do this;" or "Nothing's coming to me;" or "I can't see anything;" then the narrative may be about not being able to do, nothing coming to you, or not being able to see something. You can MT to be sure.

When you begin telling the narrative:

MT • *Am I in the right place?*

If yes, continue with story.

If no, just take a breath and set the intention to get more receptive and go back into sensation. Check the question again until you get a yes. This happens very infrequently.

If you are doing this with a partner, it's important to support them as they find the story. Say things like: *"That's right." "What is happening now?" "Yes, and . . ." "What are you experiencing next?"*

It's of critical importance that you don't "lead" the person as the story is revealed. Do not ask any questions about something in the story that you think is important, that interests you, etc.

4.4. Once you sense you have found the whole story, **MT** • *Do we have the whole narrative?*

> **If no,** go back into the body sensations to find the rest of the story until the answer to Question 4.4 is yes.
>
> **If yes,** proceed to Question 4.5.

4.5 Now that you have the complete story, it's time to do the intervention(s), if any are called for. If no interventions are called for, proceed to Question 4.6.

Allowing yourself to feel any remaining body sensations, do the intervention(s) until it feels complete.

After doing the intervention, **MT** • *Is the intervention now complete?*

> **If no,** continue with intervention until the answer to Question 4.5 is yes.
>
> **If yes,** proceed to Question 4.6.

4.6 MT–*Is the HPI now fully balanced?*

> **If yes,** proceed to Question 4.7
>
> **If no,** **MT** • *Will the intention balance on its own later?*
>
>> **If yes,** proceed to Question 4.7.
>>
>> **If no,** **MT** • *Is there another intervention to find and do?*
>>
>>> **If yes,** find and do the intervention. (You can use Questions 3.3 and 3.4 as prompts for finding this intervention.)
>>>
>>> After finding and doing the intervention, recheck for balance. You should get a yes.
>>>
>>> **If no,** check to see if a "layer" has balance. **MT** • *Is this layer fully balanced?* Answer is likely to be yes. Proceed to Question 4.7.
>>>
>>> A layer is like a chapter in a book. You've taken care of a part of the intention and there are more narratives to come.

4.7 MT • *Shall we restate the intention in the positive form?*

If yes, restate the intention in the positive form and MT the statement. Answer should be yes.

If no, proceed to Question 4.8.

4.8 *What happened to earlier sensation(s)?*

If no sensation(s) remains, proceed to Question 5.1.

If sensation(s) remain, proceed to Question 4.9.

4.9 MT • *Are any other interventions called for related to sensation(s)?*

If no, proceed to Question 4.10.

If yes, find intervention using Questions 3.3 and 3.4 and then do intervention and proceed to Question 4.10 if there is remaining sensation(s). If no sensation(s) remains, proceed to question 5.1.

4.10 MT • *Are we to dialogue with the remaining sensation(s)?*

If no, proceed to Question 4.11.

If yes, bring all attention to the sensation(s) and let it share. If any sensation(s) remains proceed to Question 4.11. If no sensation(s) remains proceed to question 5.1.

4.11 MT • *Is sensation(s) associated with another blocked intention?*

If yes, MT • *Are we to work with it now?*

    If yes, go to the beginning of the protocol and do a healing with the alleviation of the sensation being the highest priority intention.

    If no, do not work with it now.

If no, remaining sensations typically release on their own. It may take a little while to integrate on the physical level and to experience the release.

Repeat Questions 4.9, 4.10 and 4.11 until the answers to all of them is no.

STEP V: CONCLUSION: INTEGRATING THE WORK AND BRINGING IT HOME

5.1. MT • *Are there any lessons to access?* (While this can be anything, this may include how the story relates to the intention.)

> **If no,** proceed to Question 5.2.
>
> **If yes,** go inside, be receptive, and find the lesson(s). Write them down. When you think you have accessed all the lessons,
>
>> **MT •** *Are the lessons complete?* Continue until answer to this is yes and then proceed to Question 5.2.

5.2. MT • Shall we ask any of the following questions?

> **If no,** proceed to Question 5.3.
>
> **If yes,** ask the following questions:

MT • *Is there any withdrawal?*

Withdrawal means you have done such a deep piece of work that you feel unsettled. The typical way to handle this is to focus on the sensation associated with feeling unsettled and do *frontal occipital holding*, or FOH.

MT • *Are there any limitations?*

> **If yes, MT •** *Is a separate healing/intervention needed?*

A limitation is something that can make you backslide—a person, place, emotion, or event. Find the limitation (person just knows or MT possibilies). Just being aware of it may take care of the problem, other times an intervention or healing may be needed. As an example, if you associate a broken marital engagement with San Francisco, going there may cause aspects of the trauma to resurface.

MT • *Do we need to anchor the healing?*

Anchoring is a way to automatically remember the benefits of the healing.

If you are to anchor the healing, choose something you typically do (e.g., twirling your hair) and then choose to associate that with the healing so that eveytime you twirl your hair, you will think of the healing.

MT • *Do we need to* **future pace** *the healing?*

If you are to future pace, go inside and imagine and experience what life is like after doing the healing. Find the good sensation(s) associated with this new way of being, become them, and experience your new way of being as if it is already happening. Notice how your life is already different in every area affected by the healing. Do this practice until it feels familiar and automatic.

MT • *Is there any anticipatory anxiety?*

    If yes, **MT •** *Is a separate healing needed?*

    If no, **MT •** *Is an intervention needed?*

Anticipatory anxiety is a fear that the process won't work or *will work*. Most of the time, a separate healing is not required. Sometimes, one of the interventions is called for. Other times, the part that feels anxious just needs to share its anxiety. If no separate healing or intervention is called for, just invite the part that is anxious to share.

MT • *Are there any practices/ behaviors and/or habit changes to deepen and maintain the work?*

If the answer to this question is yes, you need to name the changes that need to happen and then choose to enact them in your life. If this is problematic, an intervention or healing may be needed.

5.3. MT • *Are you to affirm the balance?*

    If the answer to this question is yes, it's an invitation to make a covenant with yourself from your heart, spoken out loud, that says you are agreeing to be in relationship with yourself and Life differently because of the work that you just completed. Or, you can ask the following questions:

    Do you accept this healing for all times, levels, and dimensions?

    Do you accept full accountability and responsibility for enacting a new way of being, with all that you have learned and all of the consequences?

5.4. MT • *Deepest Wisdom, Highest Guidance, Source, is there anything else you wish to share?*

> If the answer to this is yes, focus inside and get receptive. Write down whatever additional sharing comes to you.

5.5. Just take a moment to allow gratitude for what you have experienced, healed, and learned.

> If you are working with someone else, you can invite them to share anything that has touched them about the work, anything they wish to remember, any reflections they have, and/or anything about what it was like to do the work. Alternatively, they can just sit quietly with themselves and integrate. We also invite you (or healing partner) to check with yourself at the end of every day and see if you notice a difference that has made a difference in your life around the work you have done.

INTERVENTIONS

These are the interventions we refer to in Steps Three and Four of the protocol.

Nine commonly used interventions are presented below. It's important to note that whenever you do an intervention, you want to allow yourself to feel the issue you are working on and its associated physical discomfort in the body. You do the intervention while focusing on the associated sensations. Notice how associated sensations shift when the intervention is complete.

Frontal Occipital Holding

Frontal Occipital Holding (FOH) is an all-purpose intervention that is particularly useful when we are feeling some kind of disconnection. Essentially, what it does is reconnect the frontal and the occipital lobes of the brain. Simply put, the occipital lobe is the area related to the capacity to experience our feelings and to have vision, and the frontal lobe is the area related to our capacity for executive decision-making. So, when we make the connection, we are reconnecting to our capacity to take heartfelt right action in the world.

How to Do It

Place one hand lightly on your forehead and one on the back of your head between your ears. Allow your head to move however it wants while gently supporting it.

Frontal Occipital Holding Exercise—Remember a time when you felt an inner sense of disconnection. For example, perhaps you had to make a decision, and you were overwhelmed by your feelings, so you had no sense of clarity. Alternatively, in order to make some decision, you hardened your heart. As a different kind of example, remember a time when you felt particularly overwhelmed, spaced-out, unable to focus. Notice the body sensation and do FOH and notice any change

Stress Release

Stress Release is an action that we take naturally without the need for teaching. When something is particularly stressful for us, we naturally put our hand on our forehead; if we were to pay attention, we would notice something seemingly magical—that our stress begins to lessen. Alternatively, we might remember a time from our childhood when we were feeling sick or overwhelmed and our mother, if she was attuned, would gently and lovingly put her hand on our forehead. Not only does this technique release stress, but it also invites us to experience the loving care of whatever, for us, is the comforting Divine Mother.

How to Do It

Place your hand lightly on your forehead.

Stress Release Exercise—Remember a time when you felt particularly stressed and in need of comfort. Notice the body sensation and do Stress Release and notice any change.

Fear Points

Rubbing or tapping the fear points can help us release anxiety, fears, or phobias. This intervention is particularly useful for our literal fears or any time we subjectively feel under attack.

How to Do It

Rub the fear points. They are located on the side of your forehead at the indent about an inch above where your eyebrows end.

Fear Points Exercise—Remember a time when you experienced fear. You might, for example, experience a time when you made a mistake, and you thought to yourself, *Oh God, they're going to kill me for this.* Another example for many of us might be doing a public presentation and the fear of humiliation we associate with doing a bad job. Notice any body sensations and do Fear Points and notice any change.

Anger Points

The Anger Points can help us release anger or rage. In order for us to understand what this really means, we have to distinguish between different kinds of anger. If someone does something that makes us understandably angry and we feel the anger to the appropriate degree, with the appropriate person, in the appropriate context, this is not a problem. After all, we are human. When we work with these anger/rage points, we are really talking about two other kinds of anger. The first one is when someone does something to make us angry, and we don't allow ourselves to experience it; instead, we numb it, and by doing this, to some degree, we numb ourselves. It is as though the energy of the anger never had a chance to be "metabolized." So, it is stuck in our body, energetically poisoning us. Working with the anger points helps us metabolize that stuck energy and release it, leading to a greater feeling of aliveness. The second kind of anger is when we use it as a way of not experiencing other deeper feeling states. Some of us get enraged as a way of protecting ourselves from hurt. Working with the anger points can help us release this defense to reveal the deeper and truer feeling with which we can then work.

How to Do It

Rub the anger points. They are located at the outer edge of the eye.

Anger Points Exercise—Remember a time when you experienced anger or rage that felt disproportionate to what you would have expected in that situation, or a time when you experienced nothing, when in retrospect, feelings of anger seemed to have been called for. For example, maybe your parent or spouse did something that could have made you feel incredibly angry, and you were too afraid to feel it. Alternatively, maybe they did something inconsequential, and you found yourself out of control with rage. Notice any body sensations, do Anger Points, and notice any change.

Shame Points

Shame Points help us release shame. Shame is the most insidious of all experiences. Unlike guilt, which is a judgment about what we have *done*, shame is a judgment about who we *are*. When we are experiencing shame, we experience the worst kind of humiliation and exposure, and all we wish to do is hide.

How to Do It

Rub the shame points. They are located beneath the lips in the indent above the chin.

Shame Points Exercise—Remember a time when you experienced shame. It may be a time when you let someone down when they were particularly counting on you, or when you felt like you made a fool of yourself. Notice any body sensations, and do Shame Points and notice any change.

Boundary Tapping

Boundary Tapping is used to create healthy, permeable boundaries. When we have truly healthy boundaries, we experience ourselves as captains of our own ship, being at choice as to what comes in and what goes out. When we experience boundary violations, our boundaries become too porous and/or too rigid. As a result, we let in too much or don't let in enough, and/or we let out too much, or we don't let out enough.

How to Do It

Tap on the boundary point, located midline on the sternum. It's typically just below the nipple line and, hence, under the bra strap on women. As you tap, focus on the discomfort associated with the boundary difficulty, noticing any other feelings, thoughts, and images that accompany this discomfort. As you're doing this, begin to affirm a healthy boundary. For example, "I am not affected by my mother's anger; it is hers and not mine." Or, "This is my daughter's sadness; I don't need to take it on."

You may also have to release difficulties associated with boundary violations when you experience these difficulties being stuck inside of you. What does this mean? Let's take the example above. Suppose your daughter gets very depressed, and then you get very depressed in a similar way. It doesn't even feel like it is yours. At some point, your daughter no longer feels depressed, yet you continue to experience the low-grade depression. It may well be that you have taken in her depression and have not known how to let it go. To take a more graphic example, let's suppose you were abused, and you are filled with a feeling of disgust and pollution that will not go away. In these examples, the tapping would be accompanied by something we call *feathering*. If you need to feather, feel the sadness or sense of pollution in your body, and, while you are doing the tapping on your sternum, *energetically vomit* out the sadness/disgust. Energetically vomiting means you will begin to retch but not actually vomit. The best way to start this is to begin by coughing and have it build to retching. While doing this, you would have your free hand move from the stomach area up to the mouth over and over as a way to represent and support the energetic release.

Boundary Tapping Exercise—Remember a time when you experienced that your boundaries were violated. You might, for example, consider a time when you felt taken advantage of. Experience the sense of violation in your body. Notice what sensations arise as you do this and any other experiences, feelings, images, and memories that accompany the sensation. Do Boundary Tapping, including feathering if it feels appropriate. Affirm the healthy boundary with all the new experiences, feelings, and images that accompany it; and notice any change.

Reversal Tapping

Reversal Tapping releases the anxiety, guilt, shame, and self-judgment associated with any reversed belief; a belief we know on a deeper level isn't true. It helps us become more open-minded to the possibility of self-acceptance. It teaches our mind to integrate this self-acceptance into every part of our being, and it affirms our basic lovability in the face of anything we might believe about ourselves.

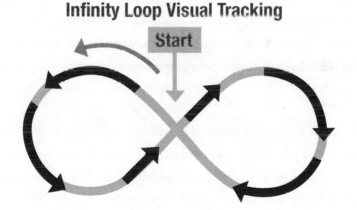

Infinity Loop Visual Tracking

How to Do It

Reversal Tapping includes three simultaneous processes: (1) Tap in semicircles around the top of your ears. (2) Have your eyes follow an infinity loop (Illustration IV) that you have drawn on a paper, or follow the corners of a wall making certain your eyes are always moving up when crossing the midline. Watch carefully to make certain your eyes do not skip. If you notice that they do skip, stay in the area that you have difficulty following. (3) While tapping and doing the eye movement, say the following repeatedly: "Even though I believe... [fill in the conflicted belief], I deeply and profoundly love, accept, and respect myself."

Reversal Tapping Exercise—Find some belief that is limiting you. There are an infinite number of possible examples. To give but a few: I am unworthy of love; I don't accept my life; I don't accept (some family member); I don't accept my body; I can't change; it's not okay for me to change; I can't heal; It is not okay for me to heal; I can't thrive, and so forth. Do Reversal Tapping and notice any change.

Letting Go

Letting Go is an intervention that facilitates the release of parts of us that no longer serve. Given that these parts have served us at one time and no longer do, it is important to thank them, and then let them go, so we have the spaciousness to open to whatever Life wishes to present next. When this is the case, this simple, powerful practice, based on Buddhist teachings, can facilitate this.

How to Do It

First, find the aspect of yourself of which it is time to let go. You can do this just by tuning into your deeper knowing. Notice any body sensations that arise. Ask this part of you how it has served and protected you. Allow yourself to send gratitude to it for all the ways it has helped you. Now, ask this same part how it has been/is limiting you. After listening to the ways it is limiting, tell this aspect it is now time to let it go. Let it go by imagining releasing it, along with the sensations and associated beliefs and feelings, through the crown of head. Experience it going to and being received by Source. Open to receiving what new gift Life has for you, confident in your knowing that it is exactly what you need for the next staging in your life. Let it fill you.

Letting Go Exercise—Find a part of you that no longer works for you in your life. It might be always being the good girl, always taking responsibility, always having to be different, always taking the contrarian point of view, always looking at the bright side—and feel this in your body. Do Letting Go and notice any change.

Light

Light can transform, balance, or integrate blocked energy. Even in our darkest hour, what we must remember is that we *are* Source and therefore are pure channels of Source energy. Source energy manifests in many ways. It can manifest as light, sound, movement, sacred symbols, and prayers.

How to Do It

First know that the Light you channel may come in a particular color or even in a rainbow. If you sense Source is coming this way, open yourself to imagining the Light bathing you and particularly infusing the discomfort in you. Often, people imagine the Light coming in through the crown of the head and filling them and then leaving through every pore of their body, taking with it all that needs to be released. Do this until you feel like everything is released or an inner Light that emanates from the deepest infinitely spacious heart expands and fills you, and you are it.

Light Exercise—Find a time when you felt overwhelmed by forces larger than yourself and when you felt too small to handle these forces, when you felt unable to care for yourself, your sense of disconnection, or your sense of not belonging. Find these sensations in your body and all the feelings, beliefs, and images that accompany them. Allow yourself for one moment to fully experience these. Then, ask Source for help. Channel Light and notice any changes.

Checking In with Yourself

After going through this protocol, we invite you to take a moment to reflect on your experience. What do you want to remember about it? What was the process like for you? How are you now compared to when you began? If you don't want to ask yourself any of these questions that's okay. We recommend you just take a little time to be with yourself before stepping back into your routine.

We invite you to check in with yourself at the end of every day to see if you notice any changes in yourself or in your life. What other things would you like to address, using this protocol in the future? We hope that you'll continue to use this protocol to heal, and if you need a helping hand, we invite you to reach out to us at www.LifeCenteredTherapy.com.

CHAPTER 15

Ending as a Beginning

There are two messages we'd like to leave you with as we come to the end of our journey. The first is that you can do this process and get miraculous results right now. We had a seventeen-year-old girl come to a weekend training. On the second day, she got matched to facilitate a very senior therapist, who looked at us as if to say, "You're sending me off with her?" We nodded. Ninety minutes later, the therapist came back and said that this was the most powerful piece of work/healing she had ever experienced. She never realized the power of letting body sensations speak for themselves, and it had never occurred to her that her problem could have originated in a karmic past life. Her young guide simply said, "I can follow a protocol."

On the other hand, we have both been guiding others for a combined fifty years and doing our own healing work as well. We are still discovering and learning new lessons every day that help us to better support our clients in their journeys. Like so many other things, you can get proficient very quickly, while capturing the true art and nuance that can add greater richness and beauty can take forever. Through using the process personally, we have achieved greater freedom, and there is a long way to go.

Even though we've been doing this work for a while, we know what it's like to be a beginner. We recognize that all of this information can seem overwhelming at first. We want you to realize that you can do this. All you have to do is find the body sensation and let it share its story. The rest of this book is just details.

When Andy went to the dentist a few weeks ago, the receptionist, Christine, commented that her allergies were terrible this year. She was dreading mowing her lawn that evening.

"Would you like me to tell you how you might get rid of your allergies?" Andy asked.

She shrugged. "Anything that can help this, I'm willing to try."

"Okay," Andy said. "Imagine that your allergies are some kind of story. What might that story be?"

She raised an eyebrow, took a moment to consider, and replied, "It seems like my body is making a mistake. It believed something was dangerous, and it had to protect itself."

"Okay. Well, while it may be true that something physical is going on, you may be living out a story that is contributing to the allergies. The story might be that you believe, for whatever reason, that the world is a dangerous place. You can't tell who is dangerous and who is safe. So, you have to protect yourself from anything that remotely reminds you of someone or something that's dangerous. Now, let yourself experience allergies and sense that the world is a dangerous place in which you can't tell who is your friend and who is your enemy. Notice what happens in your body."

Christine sneezed and sniffled, and she rubbed her eyes. "They're itchy," she said.

"Now, bring all of your awareness to the allergy symptoms and become them. And just be receptive to whatever comes to you."

Christine rubbed her nose with a tissue, closed her eyes and focused. A moment later, she opened her eyes and said, "They're going away—the allergy symptoms. Huh, interesting."

"Did you find a story?" Andy asked.

"Something came to me, but I'm not going to share it with you," she said.

"That's fine," Andy said. "I'm glad it helped."

"I'm glad my nose stopped running," Christine said, "but I doubt this will hold up when I mow the lawn later."

Two weeks later, Andy had to go back to the dentist. When Christine heard his voice, she literally ran from the back room to the front of the office.

"It's a miracle!" she exclaimed. "I did the same practice before I mowed the lawn, and then I mowed the lawn and had no allergic reaction whatsoever. And the reaction has stayed away for two weeks. It's so unbelievable. I've been telling all of my family and friends about it and telling them to do the same thing."

Christine had not read this book. All she did was focus on her symptom (allergies) and then listen to what "Allergies" needed to share with her. That's it. And her allergy symptoms went away. As we have said before, it's not always this easy, but sometimes it is.

You can do this, too. You *can*. You don't have to spend time wondering if you're doing it right—you are. You don't have to be a licensed therapist, a physician, a religious leader, or a yogi. You don't have to study more or read more or prepare more. You just need to be you—exactly as you are in this moment. And you've got to have faith in yourself—in your own wisdom. You have all you need within you now. You have the power to heal yourself. You've had the power all along. A part of you has known this all along as well because that part led you to pick up this book and bring this knowledge to your conscious mind. There's a reason—a perfectly orchestrated reason —that Life led you to this place of wisdom in this moment. It's our great hope that you will allow this book to lead you to a deeper understanding of your place in Life and of the meaning of the experiences you have in Life.

It's true that you can get miraculous symptomatic results as the title of the book, *The One-Hour Miracle*, suggests, and through these miracles,

the beginning of gaining greater meaning and freedom from the very first
session on. If most people's experience when going down this path is any
indication, the work gets harder and more arduous when your intention
moves from symptom relief to a greater freedom—the freedom from the
confines of our personality and our automatic ways of being.

We broaden our capacity to be with all that Life brings our way , knowing "I'll be okay" no matter what happens. At this point you can face any
circumstances with courage and grace, enabling you to find and maintain
a sense of inner peace. You can attune to your deepest inner knowing that
knows what is true for you and knows what you truly desire and aspire to
when you are in alignment with Life.

Then you can live a life of true aliveness and presence with all of your
wisdom, love, and full engagement. At this point, it is as if the experience
transforms alchemically from *The One-Hour Miracle* to the journey of a
lifetime, A Journey to Re-member.

We are told the French have a saying that, loosely translated, means:
"It's time for your butterflies." This may be a pivotal moment for you—a
moment to appreciate the great beauty of Life, to have greater clarity and
perspective of your place in it, and to access the wisdom that is innately
part of you that knows there is nothing to fear. Embrace it. Simply close
your eyes, focus in and down, and listen. Heal your traumas so that you
can shine—so that you can fly as effortlessly as a butterfly that has broken
through its chrysalis. Then, share your gifts and your beauty with others
as you are meant to in the ongoing mystical, magical evolution of Life.

We can't wait to hear all about it! Let us know your experiences at www.LifeCenteredTherapy.com.

Keep an eye out for our next book, *The Seven Steps to Transformation*. This next book will walk you through steps you can take when a limitation you experience isn't based on a trauma. You'll learn how to:

1. find passion and destiny;

2. release blocks;

3. master self-healing skills;

4. raise your vibration;

5. mature into a deeper level of wisdom;

6. take multiple perspectives in any situation; and

7. tap into Unity Consciousness.

APPENDIX

Here we present eight less commonly encountered patterns in the LCT healing system. Even though they don't seem to come up as often, if they do come up, they are always a significant and important part of someone's journey. We recommend that you read through these and see if any resonate with you.

Loss Trauma Pattern

I feel empty.

A Loss Pattern typically is a result of a traumatic material loss, such as losing a loved one. However, this pattern can be associated with any event in which loss is a theme, such as losing a part of oneself.

During the AIDS epidemic, I lost thirty people in three years. I turned to drugs and alcohol to mask the pain of losing so many loved ones. I worked on that pain in Life Centered Therapy and was able to get closure on the deaths of those people. A lot of my thinking that led me to substance abuse has changed. I don't have the need to use as an addict would anymore. And miraculously, I also don't have to be afraid of having one glass of wine with dinner. If I'm upset, I'm not going to have that glass of wine—I'm going to experience my feelings instead. That's a profound change for me. I've never achieved this sense of control and peace before.

This is very different from the twelve-step ideology in which you are deemed powerless and helpless—that's a very black-and-white way of thinking. I think that the twelve-step ideology programs you to think that if you slip up, it's all over. My work in Life Centered Therapy is the opposite—it's empowering. I have developed a strong sense of personal responsibility and an understanding that I'm a grown adult and that I have power and control over what I do. It works much better for me. It's a much more achievable goal for a lot of people—rather than saying that I can never have another glass of wine as long as I live, I say that I'm a grown man who can have one glass of wine and remain in control and not get drunk. I have some control over what I do.

This coming to realize my own personal power affects all areas of my life in which I've felt helpless. Through Life Centered Therapy, I'm learning more about my strengths and weaknesses, and I'm discovering that I'm a hell of a lot stronger than I thought I was. *

—G. H. Friedlander

When an individual suffers a major loss, they experience a shock on the emotional and energetic levels. Anger/rage, sadness/despair, and hurt/pain are typical responses. They may try to make sense of it or understand why it occurred with such thoughts as: the loss was my fault; people are not trustworthy and will leave; I am unlovable or unworthy; or life is vicious. In addition, they may put up walls to other relationships and/or, in reaction to emptiness, use relationships compulsively. Relationships need not just be with other people: their relationship to their behaviors, as an example, eating food, can also be affected either by not taking in enough or by eating addictively.

---

* The view expressed here is the opinion of this particular client and is not to be taken as the views of the Life Centered Therapy Institute.

A Case: Caste Away

Jane was a woman who was experiencing inexplicable depression and anxiety for the past twenty years. She had been in traditional talk therapy for the past fifteen years and taking psychiatric medication, but nothing helped. She had suicidal thoughts for much for her life, and at the age of fifteen, she attempted suicide.

She came into the session to work on her general high anxiety levels, her unexplainable anxiety around people, a feeling in her throat, an inability to express herself due to fear, and a strange feeling she had been carrying for as long as she could remember that she was going to be abandoned and left behind.

Muscle testing indicated that we were to work on all of these. In other words, all of these difficulties were all part of the same narrative and crystallized at a point in time where some set of experiences became too much for her to handle and integrate.

Muscle testing indicated that there was a Loss Pattern that was out of her awareness and key to her healing. Saying, "I feel empty," the inducting statement for a Loss Pattern, Jane began to cry and say that it all resonated so, so deeply for her.

"I don't know why I'm crying," she said. "Ever since I was small, I've felt so, so sad, and there's been no reason for it. I've carried this heavy, unexplainable grief for a long time and have overwhelming feelings all the time. I can't explain why I cry all the time. It's always felt like I've had a huge loss, but I had an okay relationship with my parents, and I had a deep understanding and acceptance when my dad died."

"I was diagnosed with depression, yet I have never felt that that was solely why I was depressed or anxious; it always felt like something deeper. I've seen therapists for more than twenty years and taken medication, but nothing helped. I've always wanted to end my life. When I had my first child, I wanted to end both of our lives as well. At the age of fifteen, I attempted suicide. I didn't know why I wanted to end my life at the time. I had an incredible childhood. I was happy all the time even with a turbulent upbringing. Then, at the age of fifteen, it just all started."

Muscle testing revealed that the root cause of the Loss Pattern was in a karmic past life. As Jane brought all her attention to, "I feel empty," and all the other experiences that were part of the loss, she felt a tightness in her throat, a tremor sensation throughout her limbs, a heaviness in her heart, and sweatiness in the palms of her hands and feet.

Speaking directly to sensations I said, "Tightness in Throat, Tremor Sensations in Limbs, Heaviness in Heart, Sweatiness in Palms and Feet, what have you come to share about loss? Where are you are beginning? What's happening?"

Jane began to cry as she told her story.

I am in India and a person of a lower caste. I was involved with someone of a higher caste. My parents disowned me because I'm pregnant . . . oh, God, I think I ended my child's life because of it. But it was for nothing because my parents never took me back. So, I ended up losing the man I loved, my parents, and the child. Oh my God! When I killed my son, I couldn't speak anymore. I don't know what happened; I just went silent. It was just a horrible, horrible situation. I couldn't speak. I was scared, anxious, sad, and abandoned. I can't tell if I ended my own life or if I was just silent for the rest of my life . . . or both. I believe I drowned.

At this point, she noticed a difference in her physical sensations. "The tightness in my throat has loosened, and my heart feels open. There is no heaviness around my heart anymore, and the tremors throughout my body have stopped . . . so has the sweating in my hands and feet."

Muscle testing indicated that we were to do an energetic intervention to finish balancing her intention and take care of the being from India whose story Jane was living out. Jane had to channel Light, and she intuited that it was a green Light to her heart and throat. After doing the intervention, she reported that she felt incredibly calm and relaxed. All the sensations and dense energies she was experiencing in her body had dissipated completely.

"For the first time in my life, I feel truly calm. I've never experienced this before; I've always been in a state of anxiety, and I thought it was normal. I feel truly different; all the sensations are gone."

The work we did was able to touch on all these different issues that might have seemed unrelated, because there was a deep structure in the form of a Loss Trauma that was foundational to all of them.

Her inability/fear to express herself that she felt in her throat was likely, on one level, a direct re-experiencing of the Indian woman who lost her capacity to speak and was silent after she killed her child, until the day she died. The unexplainable feeling that she was going to be abandoned and left behind that she had since she was young may have been a re-experiencing of the profound loss and isolation she experienced when she lost her lover, child, and family.

Her unexplainable depression that was resistant to medication and therapy for twenty years may have been due to the profound feelings of emptiness, loss, and grief she was carrying from that prior lifetime. Her desire to end her and her child's life in her current life may be a direct bleed through of her past life (or imaginal story), too.

Her feeling that, "Ever since I was small, I felt so sad, and there was no reason for it," may be explained by the fact that she was holding this Loss Trauma since she was fifteen years old in that prior life and had come into this lifetime to heal this karma, so that it was there from as early as she could remember as a way of preparing her to do this.

It appears that, since Jane's issues in her current lifetime appeared out of the blue when she was fifteen after a relatively happy childhood that couldn't account for her symptoms, turning fifteen might have been a trigger on a Soul level, as it was the exact age the Loss Trauma in her past life (or imagined story) crystallized.

This session is a great example of how working with deep structure and unconscious and universal patterns that may be out of our awareness and opening to possibilities outside of the paradigm of Western reality can impact multiple symptoms simultaneously that may be resistant to talk therapy, pharmacology, and other interventions.

The following is Jane's experience in the days after the session:

My session was truly transformative. It turns out that a past-life situation bled through to my current life, causing some emotional and mental stress. My "childhood traumas" were not the root cause of my mental anguish. Apparently, five lifetimes ago, I was born into the lower-class system in India. I met a beautiful boy who made my heart sing. And he loved me just as much as I loved him.

And you won't believe how much of that story bled through into my present incarnation. I attempted suicide at fifteen. When I carried my first child, I also contemplated ending both our lives.

All the therapy sessions, counseling, prescription drugs, and recreational drugs did not help me. I always felt as though something was wrong with me. I had such a difficult time accepting the psychological and psychiatric diagnoses assigned to me.

Since our session, I am super happy to report how much more at peace I feel around people. And my interactions are much more fluid and authentic. Also, something physically, mentally, emotionally, and spiritually has shifted. It's very challenging to use words that are so limiting.

It's as if I am someone else. The integration process was powerful and seamless. I felt some subtle, yet strong changes in my energy bodies and thought patterns.

Today was the first day I worked with a group of complete strangers and felt at ease. In the past, I would have politely declined the invitation to collaborate with teens or would have not shown up. The other thing I have observed and am witnessing is the transfiguration of my affections toward my significant other. My expressions of love, gratitude, and compassion are energetically more passionate. It's as if a veil of dullness has been lifted. It is hard to describe with words. It has been truly a life-changing experience.

Violence Trauma Pattern

I feel vulnerable./I feel polluted.

When a person experiences a Violence Trauma Pattern, they experience a shock on the emotional and energetic levels. In addition to the initial shock and fear, anger/rage, sadness/despair, and hurt/pain are typical responses. It's not uncommon that the attack results in major safety issues. The victim no longer feels capable of maintaining a personal boundary and continues to feel vulnerable. Another possible effect of this violation is a feeling of extreme shame. Sexual violence, in particular, often results in feelings of being polluted or tarnished.

Victims of violence may develop limiting beliefs in an attempt to rationalize what happened. Shame and guilt will develop if they blame themselves. The person may blame someone other than the perpetrator for not protecting them. Sometimes, the victim experiences a profound disconnection from God for allowing the trauma to happen. In addition, there may be a generalization of distrust (e.g., men are dangerous), feelings of powerlessness, a fear of power or a belief that power is bad, or a feeling of being unlovable, unwanted, or unworthy. Balancing the trauma typically simultaneously also balances these limiting beliefs, allowing the victim to place the onus of responsibility where it belongs—on the actual perpetrator.

While violence is often a random act, people who have suffered repeated acts of violence often have a set-up. For example, an initial violation may create a sense of powerlessness and an inability to maintain boundaries (whether the initial violation occurred in this or other lifetimes or imaginal stories).

People who have suffered a Violence Trauma often present with fear (phobias, flashbacks, nightmares). It may be difficult for them to develop intimate relationships, let anyone physically near them, or, in extreme cases, even to leave their homes. These fears may be accompanied by a sense of over-responsibility or victimization, an inability to feel feelings, overwhelming feelings used as a defense against real feelings, and/or boundary issues (particularly with whoever violated them—including a group association—or who ought to have protected them).

A Case: Blindsided, an Atypical Presentation of a Violence Trauma

> There is no such thing as chance,
> and what seems to us merest accident springs
> from the deepest source of destiny.
> –Friedrich Schiller

Suzy, a twenty-six-year-old woman, came in for a session because she was experiencing post-traumatic stress disorder (PTSD) and other symptoms after a car accident. In addition to flashbacks, Suzy felt constantly upset with "everything in life." She felt a nonspecific guilt, anger, and resentment toward her father for his abusive treatment of her as a child, and she was scared of everything. She also said that she was having nightmares. Muscle testing indicated that the most important thing to work on was "feeling upset about everything under the sun," and that it was equal to a Violence Trauma Pattern that occurred at age ten.

When Suzy allowed herself to fully experience, "I feel vulnerable," she immediately felt pain in her teeth, difficulty breathing, tingling in her hands, lightheadedness, and a feeling of being off-balance and tilting to her left side. As she dropped her consciousness into these sensations, she reported the following: "It feels like I was hit by my eye . . . I'm feeling cold in my face. It's slippery wherever I am, and I keep focusing on my face. I'm tipping over like I'm laying down. There is a tingling sensation on the left side of my face, and my right shoulder hurts. Now, I'm remembering being on a playground, and it's this girl's birthday.

"It's really cold out, and there is ice and snow. We were playing tag, and the bases were trees and poles. I can see myself running from the trees, turning around as I ran to see if someone was chasing me to tag me. And the second I looked forward, I hit the pole with full force, and I fell.

"I remember I lost my hearing and my vision and was knocked unconscious. When I woke up, my hands were scraped, there were some small white pieces of something in front of me, but I don't know what they were. My chest was hurting, and I was leaning to the left. I was crying.

"Oh my God; those are my teeth! I try to put one of them back in, but I swallow it. It's sharp, and it hurts. My chest feels like I've been crying; the left side of my face is tingling exactly where I hit the pole.

"I remember that I really wanted my mom. I was just so upset. I was at school, and she wasn't there for me . . . and even now, that makes me want to cry. I didn't want to cry at school, and I was just upset consistently after that.

"I'm seeing a lot of direct parallels from that experience and my car accident. When I crashed, I looked away from the wheel, and I hit a car and spun into traffic. The impact of the airbag made me lose my hearing and vision, and my face went numb. It's exactly like when I ran into the pole when I was ten, and my hearing and vision were gone. My face went numb, and I was knocked unconscious. The same thing happened both times. I'm also realizing that in both experiences, my mom was at work and not there for me. After the car accident, my mom couldn't get to the hospital, and I was alone again, just like when I was little."

Two weeks after the session, Suzy reported that she had fewer flashbacks, fewer nightmares, and no more feelings of fearing everything in her life. She was no longer getting extremely upset about minor annoyances in her life or overreacting. The change in her symptoms is indicative that working on the root-cause trauma was fundamental in healing her PTSD symptoms.

We invite you to note here that anything that makes you feel vulnerable can map as (i.e., be traced to) violence. It doesn't necessarily have to be by a person or an animal; it can be an "attack" by a pole.

Already Dead Parts Pattern

Part(s) of me is/feels numb or already dead.

Already Dead Parts are the next line in a continuum following the Death Wish. In a Death Wish, parts of us want to die/complete a death process. In an Already Dead Parts Pattern, we experience something so traumatic that, energetically, a part of us dies. We experience ourselves in this area as numb and/or hopeless. Unlike in a Death Wish where the split-off part wants to complete a death process, this already split-off dead part wants to come back to life again.

Any part of us can deaden. If our hands deaden, we may be unable to manipulate the world in the best sense of that word; if our heart deadens, we may lose our capacity for empathy and compassion; if our solar plexus deadens, we may lose our capacity to take a stand; if our sexual area deadens, we may lose our capacity for creativity, passion, and ecstasy.

This deadening response may be in reaction to tremendous fear, shame, anger, pain, or sadness that simply feels too overwhelming or threatening to experience. In this way, it is similar to the Split/Multiple Pattern we talked about before, but instead of dissociating, a part of the person gives up. An Already Dead Parts Pattern can typically manifest as hopelessness, despair, or withdrawal.

A Case: Dying to Sing

Freddie came into a session saying that he really wanted to work on his lack of passion in life. He went on to say that he felt numb most of the time, "Kinda' like feeling dead." Muscle testing revealed that this was exactly what he was to work on, and it was an Already Dead Parts Pattern.

Freddie was to begin by doing an intervention called Anger Points, which meant that he was to massage the spot directly next to his outer eyes. Explaining this intervention, I told Freddie that at some point, something happened to him that made him very angry. He did not feel safe to experience that anger, so it remained stuck in his body, unmetabolized. It was as if this stuck energy was poisoning him, preventing him from experiencing passion in life.

Just after Freddie said, "Parts of me feel already dead," he said that he had a terrible lump in his throat and felt very overwhelmed. Bringing all of his attention to the lump and letting it share, he said, "Oh my God; I'm taking speech lessons because I'm stuttering. I love to sing, and I want to join the choir. I'm asking my parents for singing lessons, and they're telling me I can't have them because they can't afford them. I feel completed deflated. I feel like a part of me died that day."

With this, Freddie began to get calmer, realizing that he had had exuberance at one time as he had recalled how much he loved singing, and as he opened to that exuberance, he could also feel all the hurt and pain of his childhood. This gave him a new perspective, and he continued: "Now I see my children, and I see how I am a different type of parent. That makes me feel so good. I feel this amazing tingling all over my body like when I listen to a song that I really love for the first time."

Freddie went on to say he felt hope for the first time in a very long time and felt capable to get through the pain. He then said, "I don't feel dead or numb at all right now. I didn't feel I deserved a good life before; now I do."

Blocked Patterns

I'm afraid if I experience (remember), I will be overwhelmed/shattered.

Blocked Patterns arise when we have an unconscious fear that if we experience or remember something, it will overwhelm, shatter, or annihilate us. It's just like the movie, *A Few Good Men*, when Tom Cruise, demands, "I want the truth;" and Jack Nicholson retorts, "You can't handle the truth." So, in a Blocked Pattern, there is always a tension—a tension between the part that believes experiencing/remembering is the only way to heal and the part that is scared to death of the experience/remembering. It doesn't reveal whether there is a literal horrific memory or just the fear there is one.

In order to protect the scared part, we create a guardian to stand watch, a sentinel whose job it is to make sure the experience/memory will never come to the surface. Just as in the tale, "The Hero of Haarlem," told in the book, *Hans Brinker, or the Silver Skates*, where the boy puts his thumb in the dike to hold back the water, so, too, the guardian tries to hold the memory at bay. As pressure builds, this invariably becomes harder and harder to do, and something seeps through. Healing arises when we care for the one who is scared so that optimal resolution becomes possible.

Interestingly, the release of the guardian does not necessarily conclude with experiencing/remembering the incident that brought the guardian forward in the first place. The client sometimes feels that it's no big deal with a "that was then; this is now," attitude. They say that they don't need to know. Sometimes it's important to remember because:

1. the perpetrator may still be a threat either to the client or others

2. there has been denial in a system of something amiss (often at the expense of the victim), or

3. the client values the truth.

A Case: A Medical Exam Draws You Out

Muriel, a woman in her mid-fifties who had been a very successful businesswoman, gave up her career success to go to graduate school so that she could become a minister. She came to therapy because one of her graduate program requirements was to get a medical exam, which included getting a blood draw. This so terrified her that she even considered giving up on going to grad school.

As we started to work on the terror she associated with a blood draw, Muriel began to have a very strange and very uncomfortable sensation in her hips. Muscle testing revealed that we needed to work directly on a Blocked Memory.

Using muscle testing, we discovered that Muriel was to bring all her attention to and become, "Very Strange and Uncomfortable Sensation in Hips." She was to let "Very Strange and Uncomfortable Sensations in Hips" share. The sensation was the beginning of the breakthrough of a potential Blocked Memory that had been held at bay by the Sentinel through numbness.

As "Very Strange and Uncomfortable Sensation in Hips" started to share, it sounded at first like it/she was saying something to the doctor. "Get away from me: you're not gonna stick that thing in me!" Suddenly, the scene changed, and Muriel was a four-year-old girl. She said that someone was at the foot of her bed, and that she was very scared. He came into the bed and started touching her and then penetrated her. It was terrifying and extremely painful, and she realized she was bleeding. At the end of the session, Muriel was able to come back to herself even though she was quite shaken. She reported that it was like she had chosen to be the four-year-old version of herself while being present and holding her.

Muriel reported that while she wasn't sure who the perpetrator was, she had a sense that it wasn't anyone she knew. She had a sense that, fifty years later, it actually didn't make any difference, and that she didn't need to know—not because she was afraid to know, but because it felt like it was just done. She also didn't remember what happened afterward when she was a little girl, although she had the sense that, for some reason, she had never shared this with anyone and quickly repressed it from her mind.

As Muriel started to reflect on her therapy experience, she had many realizations. It never would have occurred to her that her terror of having a blood draw was associated with sexual abuse she endured at age four. She had never really realized that there was something underneath why she wouldn't let anyone touch her or hug her. It just struck her that that was the way she was, and it was no big deal. It never occurred to her that it was her way of protecting herself from something that she had totally repressed.

These sessions were just the beginning of Muriel's journey that ended up with her barely being able to get the blood draw about a year later. Getting the blood draw, however, was the least important result for Muriel. This case shows all the levels LCT work affects. On a material level, Muriel was able to release levels of numbness through doing an intervention called Emotional Freedom Technique in which you tap on many accupressure meridians. She then literally was able to get the blood draw. On a symbolic level, she was able to distinguish the penetration and blood of the sexual violence with penetration of the blood draw. On a Soul level, she was able to release her need to be responsible and to control to such a degree that she was able to go to all of her professors and ask for extensions when necessary when she had previously never not done something on time. She also was able to let someone touch her. Being able to get a blood draw paled in comparison to these results for her. On a spiritual level, Muriel's ultimate conclusion was that she had chosen her true calling, and that if she was going to ask people to be with their pain, she had to fully be ready to face and be with all of hers.

Individuation Trauma Pattern

I feel separate from Source.

Individuation refers to the process in which a person develops her/his own unique identity and "leaves the nest." An Individuation Trauma Pattern occurs when something goes wrong in the separation. The separation can be from whatever is the source from which the person came, and the source will be unique to the narrative. The source can be God, our parents, or even our schoolteachers as we graduate and go into the "real world." Whatever the source that the person feels separated from in these stories, they often feel responsible for the loss of connection. When a person suffers this loss, they may succumb to some other energy, enticing them to take the place of what sourced them. If it is a separation from God story, that energy will likely be some nonmaterial form, like the devil. If it is a separation from parent story, it might be another individual that is a bad influence. Whoever the influencer, it gains power over them. If they do not succumb to another influencer, there is usually a profound sense of being alone and searching for connection.

Some people experience the process of being born and separating from their mother's body as a trauma, while others don't experience birth that way. Think about the separation anxiety a toddler feels when she toddles away from her mother to explore the world on her own, but then when she turns around and doesn't see her mother, she panics. Another good example is when a precocious teen races into a situation with boundless excitement and little regard for any potential consequence. Or, to put it differently, fools rush in where angels fear to tread. These teens can find themselves in trouble and alone, separated from their parents in a situation wherein they suddenly want their help desperately. Yet another example is when a person enters a different culture and loses his bearings. In this case, they are separate from everything that is familiar to them.

Whatever the narrative, the nature of the healing is the same: to repeat the birthing/separation process, this time doing it in a different way. Typically, how this happens is the person goes through the individuation consciously while keeping their connection with their source as they do, so that they have the subjective experience of not losing the connection when they are "born." Often this is accompanied by channeling Light from Source so that there is a sense of a band of energy maintaining the connection even while they go out and explore the world.

A Case: A Rainbow Brings You Home

Leah, a forty-five-year-old married woman, came to treatment for a general and vague sense of dissatisfaction in her life. She had mixed feelings about her marriage and experienced herself being stuck, neither able to fully commit nor to separate. While feeling good about her work as a healer/religious teacher, she sensed that she could be doing more. She described trying to will herself to be happy, affirming all the wonderful aspects of her life. But the harder she tried, the more she couldn't do it.

Muscle testing revealed that Leah was to work with an Individuation Trauma Pattern that originated when her Soul first separated from Source in this universe, and that she was to transform the pattern with rainbow Light.

Leah made the inducting statement, "I feel separate from God." A sickened, stricken look came over her face, and she cried softly, "My chest hurts so much." She could sense herself leaving the Light, and she so wanted to get into this universe to do her work as a human on Earth that she lost her sense of connection. "It's as though I don't know where I came from," she said. Leah described a sense of being profoundly lost. Then, she yelped. She said that a strange, birdlike creature was coming to her. "I'll take care of you" it said enticingly. She felt it getting into her body so that while she was experiencing a sense of emptiness, she also sensed this energy within her. Yet, when she tried to focus on it, it was hard to find. She said that it felt like she was cursed, and that she would never be able to find God again. "I've been on my own [separated from God] for such a long time," Leah said. "I've only had myself to count on."

I suggested to her that, even though she felt that she had lost God, God was still here. I invited her to amplify both the sense of emptiness and the sense of this birdlike creature that was within her. She could do both simultaneously and said that the emptiness felt too big for her, and that she couldn't fight the creature anymore, who felt like it was ripping up her insides. She now had the whole story and started channeling the rainbow Light. I reminded her that God was bigger than the emptiness and the creature. She responded, "No, there is no rainbow Light. I'm not loved by God." She started crying.

Shortly thereafter, her face started to change, and the tears seemed calm rather than agitating. She softly said, "The rainbow Light is starting to come. I couldn't will it to come; I just feel like I'm receiving it." She sat for a while quietly, and then looked up, "The creature is gone. My emptiness feels full." She said that her heart felt like it was full of love, and that there was no more pain.

There were lessons for Leah. She said, "I've been such a controlling person. I even tried to control this healing. It was like I was trying to use my mind to stop the healing. Yet, the rainbow Light was stronger than my will. My mind was saying, 'This is impossible,' but I can feel now that there is something bigger than my will. I have some inner sense that I'm going to stop fighting now." The key for Leah was to reconnect with Source/God, which she did by opening up to the rainbow Light and allowing it (Source/

God) in. This healed her Individuation Trauma (her trauma of feeling separate from Source/God).

Six years later, Leah, reflecting on the session, said, "Up until that session, I had a profound sense of being bad. I tried to will myself to overcome it and be good, and it never worked. After that session, inexplicably this feeling started to leave my life on its own. It's like I became more acceptable and more accepting, and I started to trust more in God's love."

Fear of Loss of Self in Relationship Pattern

I am unable to handle the anxiety that accompanies being in a relationship with you. Therefore, I defuse the anxiety by sabotaging by (choose all that apply): compulsively making myself too distant, making myself too close, going on automatic in the relationship, or bringing in something else (person or thing).

A Fear of Loss of Self in Relationship Pattern occurs when a person is unable to handle the anxiety in their relationship with another person or any system, meaning within a family, a work group, or in a church congregation for example, and therefore sabotages it to defuse the anxiety.

To be in a true I/Thou relationship with another asks for a deep level of maturity, responsibility, and integrity. A mature relationship also calls for a high degree of communion and autonomy. A wonderful explanation of communion and autonomy is expressed beautifully in an excerpt from Kahlil Gibran's poem, "On Marriage:"

> *Love one another, but make not a bond*
> *of love:*
> *Let it rather be a moving sea between*
> *the shores of your souls.*
> *Fill each other's cup but drink not from*
> *one cup.*
> *Give one another of your bread but eat*

not from the same loaf.
      Sing and dance together and be joyous,
but let each one of you be alone,
      Even as the strings of a lute are alone
though they quiver with the same music.
      Give your hearts, but not into each
other's keeping.
      For only the hand of Life can contain
your hearts.
      And stand together yet not too near
together:
      For the pillars of the temple stand apart,
      And the oak tree and the cypress grow
not in each other's shadow.

When we are unable to maintain such communion and autonomy, and the fear of the loss of self surfaces, this can change the way we act in relationship, and we can lose our capacity for true connection. We might become too enmeshed, too isolated, or both.

Loss of Self in Relationship: Triangular Version

The triangular version of this pattern comes into play when we are struggling with a relationship with another person because the relationship itself is creating anxiety for us. So, we unconsciously bring in some other person and/or experience to deflect or avoid that anxiety. It's just like bringing in a buffer.

A Case: Choosing to Give Life

Steve, who is writing a book with a woman named Jane, came to therapy. He reported that he was feeling torn between his life work and writing the book with Jane, versus creating enough time to be with his wife and for other things. He felt like his wife was putting a lot of pressure on him that he was having a great deal of difficulty not just caving in to. He felt a little bit like he was being torn apart. Then, he said, almost as an afterthought, "I had a very strange experience this morning. I was looking intently in the mirror, and I saw myself begin to change shape. My face started to become different and looked like a woman, and then I had a sense that she was looking back at me wearing Roman garb."

Muscle testing revealed that this woman was the central character in the story he glimpsed in the mirror. Just hearing this, Steve began to shake. Bringing all of his attention to a shaking sensation, he said:

> *I know what's happening. I am the woman I saw this morning. I am pregnant, in fact. He's been controlling me all along, and now he is pressuring me to get an abortion. He doesn't want that responsibility, and he wants me all for himself.*
>
> *I can't believe it. I'm caving into the pressure, and I'm actually having the abortion. I am hating myself for this, and I'm hating him. And I'm just too weak to stand up for myself. I've got to learn this lesson. I don't want to ever let anyone have this much power over me again. I truly want to have this baby, and I let him get in the way. I didn't have the courage to stand up for myself. Maybe the baby would've been a way to have gotten away from my relationship with my husband. I'm realizing that, not only did I want to have the baby, I wanted to have the baby as a buffer. So, he was probably right; he wouldn't have me all to himself. And the irony is that he didn't have that in the first place. But of course, I didn't have myself either.*

As soon as Steve said this, somethings shifted. It's like his whole body relaxed, and the shaking, which had been pronounced, just stopped. Steve said that he suddenly felt a strong need to protect his writing time "as if it were my child." Then he said, "I get it. The book is my baby, so to speak. And my wife is the controlling husband in the story. I can't let this pattern continue."

Steve went home with resolve and informed his wife that he would be prioritizing the book until it was completed. Then, he called his writing partner and pledged to remain steadfast in his dedication to completing the book. He made good on that pledge, and the two finished the book before the deadline.

Seduction Pattern

To feel alive, I seduce others. / To feel alive, I let others seduce me.

Let's now turn to the Seduction Pattern. Seduction Patterns are generally associated with a person not feeling fully alive and therefore connecting inappropriately with others in order to feel a kind of pseudo-aliveness. While the overt behavior may be sexual in nature, it really has to do with a compulsion to connect. These kinds of inappropriate connections lead to unhealthy attachments and codependent relationships.

Seduction can show up in two ways. We can be the one who is seduced, or we can be the one who is the seducer. The pattern can play out in two realms—material and/or nonmaterial. An example in the material realm would be a mother–child relationship in which the mother is depressed. The child defers to the mother's need in order to reanimate the mother, and so the child does anything it can (essentially trying to seduce the mother) to get responsiveness from her so that the sense of attachment can be experienced again. The mother, in turn, lets herself be seduced as a way of having a sense of inner aliveness. Thus, the two are not involved in a healthy I/Thou relationship but an I/It relationship. An I/Thou relationship is one of mutuality and respect for the other for who they are; an I/It relationship is characterized by objectification of the other to meet one's needs.

In the nonmaterial realms, an example might be the German legend of Faust and Mephistopheles. Faust, having an inner sense of lack, called in the devil to have a sense of omnipotence. The devil, needing to obtain Souls, agreed to the request on the condition that Faust would sell his Soul. Once again, we can see both the I/It nature of the relationship and the forming of a relationship from an inner sense of lacking.

To transform the Seduction Pattern, we must feel our inner sense of lack and unfulfillment, and experience, allow, and accept the parts of us that feel numb. By refusing the fool's gold that we get on either side of the arrangement and instead opening ourselves to Life/Source, we can receive the real thing and can experience a true sense of inner fulfillment.

A Case: Feeling Alive at All Costs

Clarisse is a twenty-seven-year-old unmarried woman who lives alone and is an only child. She seemed subdued but not depressed. She came in for a session, saying that she felt an impending sense of harm—that something bad would happen.

"Nothing ever works out right anywhere," she said. "I have this anger that randomly shows up, and I don't know why. No one ever really chooses me, and I don't feel like I choose anything." She went on to say, "I'm the one who does all the birthday parties for my friends, and I feel if I didn't do things like this for them, they would all go away. While it seems like people like me, I don't believe that they really do."

Muscle testing revealed she was not to work on any of these; she was to work on a Seduction Pattern in which she was the seducer. When she said, "I seduce others in order to feel alive," she immediately felt an emptiness and hurt in her chest. She started to sweat, and she said, "They're burning people; it's a funeral. They are going to burn me alive. I feel paralyzed. I'm not able to say, 'But I'm not dead.' Oh, my God. It's where they killed men's wives after the men have died. Oh God, it's so hot."

She stopped, and then she said, "I gave up my son to be in a harem because when my husband died, I thought it was a way to survive and not be killed. In order to be in the harem, I had to let my son go to the streets. In the harem, I felt like property. There was no connection and no status for me. When the harem dissolved because the second man in my life died, I was facing death again. I have a sense I was duped . . . doubly duped.

Being in the harem didn't bring me safety and was less than what I thought it would be." She laughed out loud. "It's like the joke about the restaurant. The food is bad *and* the portions are too small. I felt a lot of anger."

Muscle testing revealed that, while she had the full content of the story, she had not revealed how she was the seducer. "Oh, oh, oh, oh," she said as tears ran down her face. "There's such a sense of pain. I told my son it was all going to be okay. I told him: 'I will come back and get you.' But I knew that wasn't true. I was seducing him into detaching. I didn't want to be with him and take care of him; I wanted to seduce the man in the harem so I could feel cared for and loved, and I couldn't do that with a son to care for." She looked up and said, "That's it."

Clarisse got very thoughtful and began to make connections between the story and her present life. She felt that it explained why she has never felt chosen, so she could begin to know what it was like for the son she did not choose and why she felt she had to do things for people to be able to stay in relationship with them, seducing her second husband so that she would feel cared for. She went on to say, "Wouldn't you feel angry if you were going to be burnt alive?" Quizzically, she asked, "How do I change all this?"

Muscle testing revealed that just finding the story was sufficient. As I was muscle testing this, she looked out the window and saw a white crow and said, "It's here for a reason." Looking up the symbolic reference, we found that crows speak to the part of us that believes, "It's better to rule in hell than to serve in heaven," which truly describes the Seduction Pattern.

Some weeks later, Clarise reported she had noticed a decrease in her general level of anger at work and had begun to wait for her friends to call her now. She admitted that this was hard to do but felt encouraged when they did call. This change alone was beginning to have a positive effect on her overall sense of self-esteem and connection in the world.

In another story, Pauline found herself in an unhealthy relationship with a Seduction Pattern at play. She needed to break the pattern to move on to a better relationship.

I was in a very tumultuous relationship of over eleven years with a man I'm wildly attracted to, but who is both adoring and emotionally and verbally abusive. He couldn't have a relationship like I wanted and share our lives together. He's a renegade. The attraction is off the charts. I don't have a strong sense of family. He kept me from feeling alone. We'd see each other once a week but talk every night on the phone. Then, we wouldn't see each other for two months. There was even a period of over two years when we didn't have sex. He didn't meet my needs physically or sexually. I moved to LA, and I still stayed with him in a relationship on the phone because I was lonely.

I tried to meet other men, but I'd still come home and talk to him at night—he was my security blanket. Being home alone at night with nobody there was very hard for me. When I was home alone at night and waiting for him to call, I'd get a sensation in my body like I was drowning, and everything was blackness. I'd feel like I was in an ocean of blackness, and there was nothing to hold onto. When the phone would ring, it was as if someone threw me a life raft. I finally had a connection with a human being who loved me. That connection helped me to feel like I wasn't going to die. I couldn't leave him and be at home alone.

Rather than talk from my mind, I was encouraged to get in touch with the sensations around my body around the fear of being alone at night. I felt like I was drowning or going to die. There was a tightness in my solar plexus and a feeling like I couldn't breathe. There was also a tightness in my chest. Then, I started to see a story unfold in my mind. When you tell these stories, who knows if they're true? But the feelings never lie, and the body knows the truth. Whether it was coming from my mind or elsewhere, I told a story of having been on a boat with some people I was connected to. I fell off the boat at night and drifted enough of a distance away that when I screamed, they couldn't hear me. I was drowning, and I drowned.

That's an example of how the body can tell a story that the mind can't even really make sense of. The feelings that come up when you're telling that story—the feelings are so potent and powerful. Somehow, becoming conscious of what you are describing and conscious of where those feelings are coming from dissipates the charge.

Within five weeks, I told that boyfriend that I couldn't talk with him anymore. Just five weeks after that, I met the man who feels like my soul mate. We're moving in together later this month.

—Pauline M.

Pauline allowed the boyfriend to seduce and control her for so long because she wanted connection and to not be alone. She literally felt like she would drown if she didn't get that human connection at night. The boyfriend seduced her to feel a sense of power and control, which she gave him in return for the company, even though it wasn't good company. With this understanding, she was able to break this pattern and break up with the boyfriend for good.

Wonderful Pattern

I long for what I've had. I compulsively seek to recreate it, destroying what I have.

A Wonderful Pattern occurs when a person has an experience that is "too good" for them to integrate into their lives. So, consciously or unconsciously, they try to recreate it/relive it. The problem is that nothing can or ever will compare to the original experience, which has been idealized to such a degree that current reality can't ever live up to it. In Wonderful Patterns, we have what is called a *positive emotional charge*. Nonetheless, it takes on the same structure as any other trauma. Anything that looks like the original situation retriggers the idealized past, and we unconsciously try to recreate it, leading to dissatisfaction and deepening craving. As with any other traumatized pattern, the key is to go back to the original situation and change our relationship with it so we can fully acknowledge and appreciate it for how special it was to us. Then, we let it go so that we can live fully in the present moment.

Vignette: Catching Glory

A classic example of a Wonderful Pattern is the old man at a bar who, as a high school football player, experienced a great moment where he caught a touchdown pass in the championship game. He can never really let it go but keeps talking about it in a vain attempt to recapture the glory which he hadn't experienced in his life since.

Vignette: The Aliveness of War

In another example, a man was experiencing ongoing, low-grade depression. This depression turned out to equal a Wonderful Pattern that originated when he was a soldier in battle. When he brought all his attention to the sensation and became it, he found himself back in a battle scene where there was great danger. As he shared the experience, he realized that it was the time in his life when he felt most alive, both because of the life-and-death nature of the event and because of the extreme camaraderie he felt with his fellow soldiers who were all in it together.

He realized that he unconsciously felt that the rest of his life was relatively mundane and insignificant. He realized that he was comparing his relationship, his work life, and his life purpose to the time he was a soldier in the war. His current relationships didn't seem as intense, the sense of being in something together was never as powerful, and the sense of working toward a common goal that gave greater meaning to everybody involved was something he was never able to recreate. This realization allowed him to begin to appreciate what truly was good in his present life and to not minimize the painful aspects about the shared war experience. He now could have a more balanced view about each.

Vignette: Carrying a Flame

A woman came in complaining that she would find relationships that looked like they would be ideal and then, seemingly for no reason, she became dissatisfied and ended them. A key moment in changing this repeating theme occurred when she found a Wonderful Pattern and realized that she was still "carrying a flame" for her first high school sweetheart. The high school sweetheart promised that they'd stay together when he moved away, but he didn't–he never contacted her again. She had idealized the relationship to such an extent that she had forgotten that he had ghosted her. By working with the Wonderful Pattern, she was able to "hold" the relationship and all that had happened appropriately. This had a very positive effect on her dating life.

Vignette: Food as Reward

Let's look at a case where a man came in, saying that his eating was out of control. He couldn't figure out why this was happening or how to stop it. Early in the treatment, his eating difficulties started to transform when we found a Wonderful Pattern. His parents were strict when it came to his eating. Yet, whenever he had an accomplishment, they would reward him with his favorite sweets. He hadn't made the connection that whenever he started to be successful, he would reward himself by binging on sweets. Shifting this experience in the body had an effect on his "out of control" eating behavior.

ABOUT THE AUTHORS

Andrew H. Hahn, PsyD

As I reflect on my life, I'm aware that I've had four ruling passions: to understand everything I can about Life, to understand relationship, to help end suffering, and to love people. All of these changed dramatically in one moment in 1991.

I was visiting a dear friend of mine named Roshan at the Self-Realization Fellowship. Roshan had fallen the day before I arrived, and her ankle was swollen, discolored, and very painful. Nonetheless, she was determined to show me the holy grounds. While we were there, her pain became so severe that she said I would have to carry her out. We both sat down, and I was suddenly flooded with extraordinary Light. I knew it wasn't the sun because I knew where the sun was in the sky, and this Light was coming from a different place. I asked Roshan to give me her ankle, and I witnessed Light going through my crown, into the center of my chest and out through my hands to her ankle. After a short time, I sensed the process was complete. Then, we looked down at her ankle. All the swelling and discoloration were gone. She stood up, walked, and didn't feel any pain; and in that moment I knew, "I wasn't in Kansas anymore." I realized how truly miraculous Life is in a way that was life-changing for me. It revealed and opened me to an idea of healing that was profoundly different from anything I'd been taught in my traditional education.

From that moment, I initiated a two-year odyssey to understand and deepen what had happened to me in that one moment. I started exploring worlds that I had not anticipated finding. I felt called to find a way to marry my traditional education in psychology with the realizations I was having about this powerful energetic and spiritual new world of healing. I knew in my heart that my role was to be a bridge between the worlds in the service of deepening our understanding, improving relationships, and finding new ways of alleviating suffering.

I'm writing this book from a place of dedication. I feel committed to sharing a framework for healing and growth that seems far simpler and more powerful, effective, and efficient than anything I could have dreamed possible when I was in graduate school or even when I was the training director in a clinic. Early in my career as a psychologist, I just knew that, though I had good tools, there had to be something more to help end people's suffering. From both my personal experience and work with hundreds of clients, I know now we have the tools I sought. We share them with you in the hopes that you will use them for your own healing and to find meaning in all that you encounter in your life.

I have been graced to be able to work with people in a new and integrated way for the last thirty years. The work keeps evolving, getting richer and simpler. I feel like the luckiest man in the world because I get to accompany people on their journeys of healing and growing that do seem truly miraculous in every hour, no matter what that hour brings. I so want to thank you for taking this journey with us.

Joan T. Beckett, LMHC, MBA

I have always been profoundly interested in people and in what makes them tick. It's always seemed that people like to share their stories with me, and I'm most interested in listening. While my undergraduate degree in chemical engineering didn't provide me with a format to formally pursue this interest, lucky me that it was easy to find opportunities in everyday interactions to hear what was happening in people's lives and to offer my interpretations if welcomed. On the technical side, I enjoyed making medicines and felt like I was contributing to making the world a healthier place. Ten years into my career, I felt blessed to be able to have the opportunity to stay at home with the two little, crack-my-heart-open-like-no-other loves of my life, David and Alexandra, fully expecting to return to big pharma when the time was right.

The time was never right. In 1998, I discovered the Life Centered Therapy training program and the Enneagram and entered the new millennium with a new way of looking at Life, a new way of looking at people, and probably most importantly, a new way of looking at and understanding myself. I was spurred on to round out my learning and received a master's degree in counselling and got myself licensed. Utilizing all the elements of left-brain training in logic and planful analysis, I partnered with Andy to tighten the thinking and clarify the philosophical underpinnings of LCT and to refine the elements of the training programs that we offer. It has been a growthful experience to marry my skill set with right-brain thinking that welcomes and supports intuition, creativity, and metaphorical understanding.

Writing the book has been a true act of love because I've seen firsthand the alleviation of suffering that results from this novel approach to "therapy." Privileged to work with courageous people who want a better life, I witness the benefit of the work every day in my practice. But to me, the message we are delivering is so much more than the problem solving we are offering. Most importantly, it is an invitation to understand our challenges in the context of meaning making and, even in our darkest hours, to have faith that a greater plan is unfolding. Our job is to learn the lessons that are being offered to us if we just look deeply enough. I feel honored that you have taken the journey through this book with us. I still love people's stories and look forward to hearing yours.